W9-BHE-355

Practical Solutions for Back Pain Relief

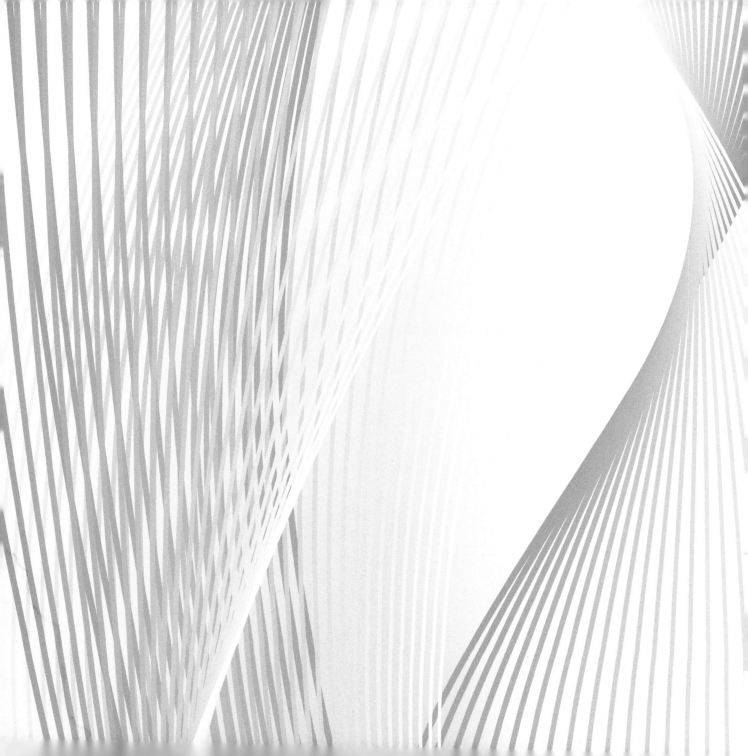

Practical Solutions for Back Pain Relief

40 BODY AND MIND EXERCISES TO MOVE BETTER, FEEL BETTER, AND RELIEVE PAIN PERMANENTLY

Dana Santas, CSCS, E-RYT

ALTHEA
PRESS

Copyright © 2018 by Dana Santas

No part of this publication may be reproduced, stored in a retrieval system or transmitted in any form or by any means, electronic, mechanical, photocopying, recording, scanning or otherwise, except as permitted under Sections 107 or 108 of the 1976 United States Copyright Act, without the prior written permission of the Publisher. Requests to the Publisher for permission should be addressed to the Permissions Department, Althea Press, 6005 Shellmound St, Suite 175, Emeryville, CA 94608.

Limit of Liability/Disclaimer of Warranty: The Publisher and the author make no representations or warranties with respect to the accuracy or completeness of the contents of this work and specifically disclaim all warranties, including without limitation warranties of fitness for a particular purpose. No warranty may be created or extended by sales or promotional materials. The advice and strategies contained herein may not be suitable for every situation. This work is sold with the understanding that the Publisher is not engaged in rendering medical, legal, or other professional advice or services. If professional assistance is required, the services of a competent professional person should be sought. Neither the Publisher nor the author shall be liable for damages arising herefrom. The fact that an individual, organization, or website is referred to in this work as a citation and/or potential source of further information does not mean that the author or the Publisher endorses the information the individual, organization, or website may provide or recommendations they/it may make. Further, readers should be aware that websites listed in this work may have changed or disappeared between when this work was written and when it is read.

For general information on our other products and services or to obtain technical support, please contact our Customer Care Department within the United States at (866) 744-2665, or outside the United States at (510) 253-0500.

Althea Press publishes its books in a variety of electronic and print formats. Some content that appears in print may not be available in electronic books, and vice versa.

TRADEMARKS: Althea Press and the Althea Press logo are trademarks or registered trademarks of Callisto Media Inc. and/or its affiliates, in the United States and other countries, and may not be used without written permission. All other trademarks are the property of their respective owners. Althea Press is not associated with any product or vendor mentioned in this book.

Author photograph © Rich Montalbano/RiMo Photo

ISBN: Print 978-1-93975-434-9
eBook 978-1-93975-435-6

This book is dedicated to everyone
who has suffered or is suffering with back pain.

I wrote this for you—to empower you to move better, feel better,
and never feel powerless against pain again.

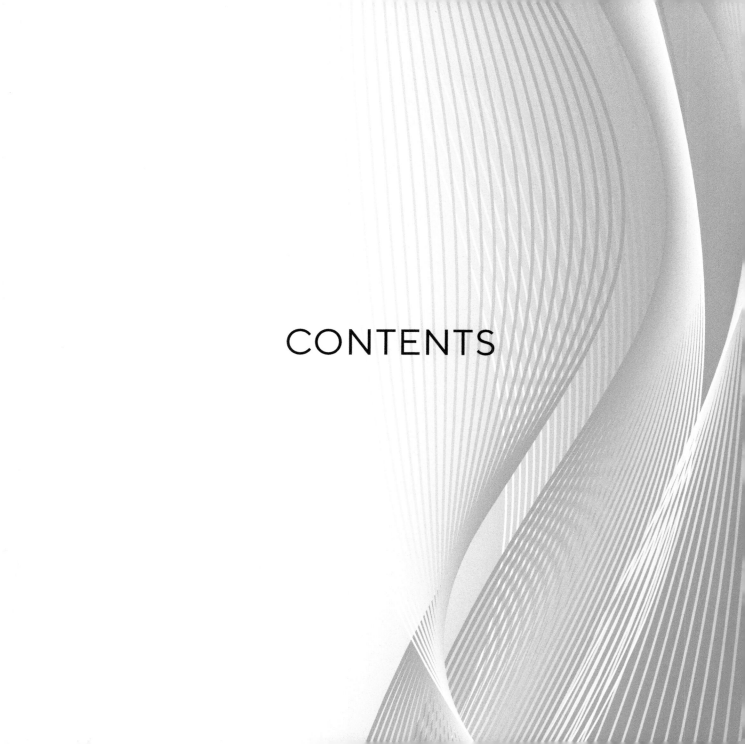

CONTENTS

Introduction   xi

Part One: Back Pain Basics   1

Chapter 1: Why Your Back Hurts   3

Chapter 2: The New Exercise Program   18

Part Two: The Exercises   28

Chapter 3: Exercises to Relieve Pain   34

›› Phase One   36

Diaphragmatic Breathing with Legs Elevated   37

Legs Up the Wall   39

Child's Pose   41

Seated Figure-Four Hip Opener   43

Supported Warrior Hip Flexor Stretch   45

Supported Back-Release Squat   47

›› Phase Two   48

Breathing Bridge on Chair   49

Kneeling Lunge   51

Gate Pose   53

Cat Flow   55

Supine Figure-Four Stretch   57

Child's Pose with Reach   59

›› **Mind-Body Exercises**   60

10-Breath Breathing Break   61

Progressive Muscle Relaxation   63

20-Breath Backward Count for Sleep   65

Chapter 4: Exercises to Regain Strength and Mobility   66

›› **Phase One**   68

Breathing Bridge   69

Sphinx with Head Turns   71

Roll-Into-a-Ball Core Exercise   73

Cobra   75

Seated Bent-Knee Twist   77

Bent-Knee Down Dog with Pedal Out   79

Standing Side Bend   81

Supine Double Bent-Knee Twist   83

Supine Figure-Four Twist   85

Bent-Knee Straddle Stretch   87

›› **Phase Two**   88

Flowing Bridge   89

Windmill Twist   91

Segmented Forearm Plank   93

Side Forearm Plank   95

Locust   97

Kneeling Lunge with Reach   99

90/90 Seated Twist   101

Pigeon   103

Seated Hamstring and Hip Stretch   105

➤➤ **Mind-Body Exercises   106**

Seated Posture Exercise with 10-Breath Breathing Break   107

Chapter 5: Exercises for Maintenance and Prevention   108

Breathing Bridge   111

Walking with Awareness of Gait Mechanics   113

Warrior Hip Flexor Stretch   117

Supine Single-Leg, Bent-Knee Twist   119

Flowing Chair Squat   121

Cat Flow   123

Supported Back-Release Squat   125

Legs Up the Wall   127

➤➤ **Mind-Body Exercises   128**

Seated Posture Exercise with 10-Breath Breathing Break   129

Compassion Meditation   131

Chapter 6: Additional Therapies for Back Pain   134

Resources   143

References   144

Index   147

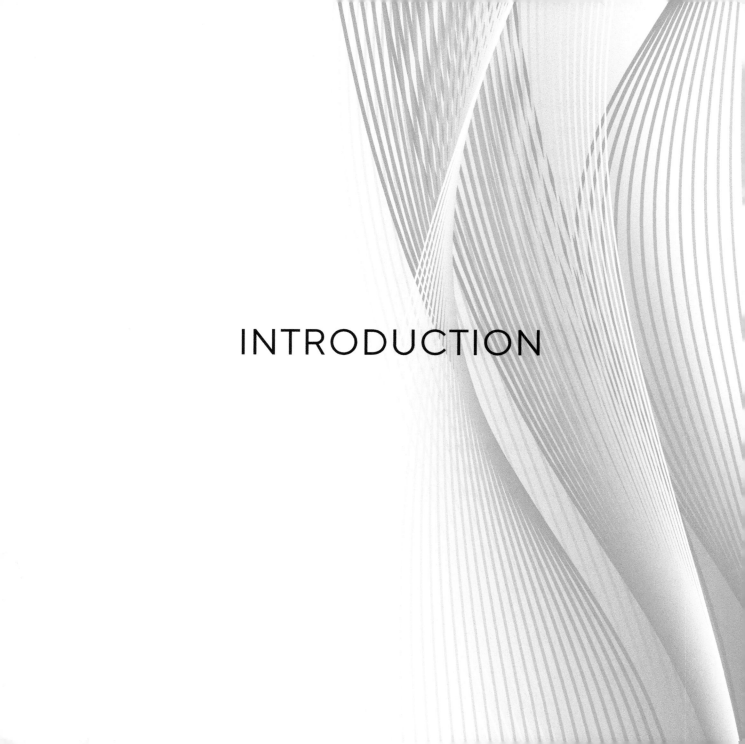

INTRODUCTION

As the "Mobility Maker," a mind-body coach in professional sports, I'm probably one of the last people anyone would expect to have suffered from back pain. In fact, teams and athletes often hire me to create programs for alleviating and preventing back pain.

Yet, like you, and the other 80 percent of the population who has suffered from back issues, I've felt your pain. I know what it's like to hurt so much that you question if you'll ever be able to perform everyday tasks pain-free, like bending down to tie your shoes or picking up your child. You are not alone. According to a recent *Consumer Reports* survey, one in four people have had an episode of back pain that severely interfered with their daily life.

For the athletes reading this, I'm also familiar with the performance-hampering anxiety—even depression—you must overcome after a back injury to return to play. The treatment and prevention of back pain is not only a large part of my career, it's also personal. My experience from both perspectives has enabled me to identify the most efficient and effective ways to relieve current,

and prevent future, back pain. As a result, this book includes easy-to-follow, practical solutions designed to empower readers experiencing back pain to take a proactive approach to relief.

But before I jump right into the solutions, you might be wondering how I ended up with back pain. That's a fair question. As I discuss in greater detail in chapter 1, back pain can have numerous causes, from a traumatic event or illness to simply feeling that we "moved wrong." And those of us who've experienced a serious bout of back pain are 80 percent more likely to experience another. I am no exception. The first time I experienced an acute back issue was in my mid-twenties. At the time I worked in corporate America, and, like many stressed-out workers, I turned to yoga. Although I'd spent several sedentary years behind a desk and hadn't exercised regularly since I was a high school gymnast, my ego believed I could jump into advanced yoga practice because of my previous athletic background. Consequently, after a couple of months forcing extreme backbends and twists I hadn't done in over a decade, I herniated two lumbar discs.

I want to be clear that *yoga did not hurt me.* *I hurt myself* by leading with my ego and not listening to my body. I went full throttle into the physical practice of yoga without working on the mind-body connection aspect, which research shows is a beneficial—if not the most beneficial—part of any yoga practice.

Because I didn't know then what I know now (and you will learn from this book), I believed my only course of action was to take the Vicodin my doctor prescribed and passively wait until the pain subsided and my mobility returned. But after about ten days of going stir-crazy in bed, and still in pain, I instinctively felt I needed to do something to help my body heal and help me get back to my life.

As counterintuitive as it seemed to return to the "scene of the crime," I went back to my yoga mat. But this time I practiced only gentle movements and meditative techniques to help me regain a sense of body awareness and reduce the fear and stress I was experiencing in response to the pain. After only a few sessions, with an increased mind-body connection and decreased pain, I was able to progress my exercises over a

month until I was finally pain-free. Unsurprising to me, a study published in *JAMA: The Journal of the American Medical Association* in 2016 found that mindfulness-based stress reduction techniques are more effective at relieving pain and restoring function than pain medication.

As horrible as it was to hurt my back, it was undeniably a valuable, life-changing experience. I was inspired to learn more about the profoundly effective mind and body exercises that enabled me to feel better and that eventually led to my career as the "Mobility Maker" in pro sports, my role as the yoga expert for CNN, and, of course, the author of this book.

All of that said, sometimes, even when we know better, we still make painful mistakes. That's exactly what happened when I reinjured my back two years ago, 14 years after the first incident. By then, having spent more than a decade working in pro sports as a mind-body coach as well as a certified strength and conditioning specialist, my own exercise program had evolved to include weight training. My favorite weight-training exercise was, and still is, the deadlift—bending over a heavily weighted bar and using a hip-hinging movement to lift it. Weighing in at 105 pounds, I was quite proud of my ability to lift 210 pounds, double my body weight.

Like my yoga practice, weight lifting had become an additional means for me to reconnect body and mind, and, when necessary, blow off steam. The day in question was one of those blow-off-steam days. Unfortunately, I let the stress of the day overpower my mind-body connection, so my ego took over without any awareness of my body's limitations. *Sound familiar?* I went too heavy, too fast, attempting to lift a significant amount of weight without proper preparation or technique. As a result, I ended up rounding my back and pulled my lumbar spine at the site of the original injury.

Again, just like my prior injury while doing yoga, I want to emphasize that *deadlifting* did not hurt my back. *I hurt myself* by leading with my ego and not listening to my body.

Sure enough, the MRI revealed bulging, herniated discs in the same place: L4, L5. But this time, even though repeating a mistake led to a second injury, I didn't make the same mistakes in my recovery. I sought out one of my professional sports teams' orthopedic doctors, who I knew favored a more progressive, noninvasive approach. We used drug-free, hands-on therapies, like acupuncture and therapeutic massage (techniques I discuss in chapter 6), to ease my pain and release muscle tension so I could begin practicing pain-relieving and strengthening movements (like the ones featured in chapters 3 and 4) on my own. Despite the acute nature of my injury, in less than a week, I was pain-free; four weeks later, I was back to training normally, and with a stronger body awareness than ever.

Although I am in the majority as someone who has experienced two significant episodes of back pain, I am in the minority as someone who has fully recovered and lives a pain-free, active lifestyle. Unfortunately, too many people suffer with chronic back pain. Because back pain tends to first immobilize you—literally leaving you laid out on the floor—and then persist for weeks, people are often so traumatized by the debilitating experience that they're willing to accept any level of improvement that enables them to function at all.

It's estimated that one in seven adults has dealt with a back pain episode that lasted at least two weeks. After putting their lives on hold to rest in bed, usually on strong pain medication, many people succumb to the pressure of their responsibilities and decide they feel "good enough," even if it means living a less-active lifestyle in chronic discomfort. Worse yet, too many of them ultimately end up with a dangerous dependency on pain medication.

Because a large percentage of the population suffers needlessly from back pain, it seems we've become desensitized to it. "Oh, my aching back" is such a commonly used phrase that it's generally accepted as a sign that a person simply needs to pop a pill. It's especially true when anyone over 50 utters that phrase. There's an assumption that your back "goes out" with age, so living with pain is a normal part of life.

But that isn't true at all! With an increasing prevalence of back pain across all age-groups, including adolescents, back pain is not a "normal" aging problem. Nor is it possible to live a "normal" life in chronic pain or while addicted to pain medication.

Living with pain is more than merely a physical deficit. Living with pain is frustrating and depressing. It has an undeniable negative impact on emotional health and perspective on life. Studies abound linking chronic pain and depression. Forget rose-colored glasses; imagine how the world looks while wearing pain-colored glasses. Maybe you don't need to imagine. And if that's the case, I am so happy you're reading this. I've written this book for you—and others like you—to empower us all with the knowledge and means to proactively live happily and pain-free.

Through an extensive review of 21 different back pain studies, *JAMA: The Journal of the American Medical Association* found that the proactive use of exercise, especially in combination with educating patients, is more effective at relieving back pain than passive methods like rest, medication, and orthotics. In fact, rest, which is the most commonly prescribed nondrug, noninvasive back pain treatment, can actually hinder recovery if it leads to prolonged inactivity. Our bodies are designed for movement. When we are inactive for long periods of time, our muscles weaken, connective tissue stiffens, and joint lubrication, including the cushioning between discs, is reduced. This not only delays healing but also increases future risk of injury.

This book is all about empowering you with a better understanding of your body's needs and how to proactively take care of them. To that end, I've included exercises that not only emphasize forging a mind-body connection but also focus on building the strength and flexibility necessary to support healthy, pain-free movement throughout your spine. Above and beyond permanently alleviating and preventing back pain, additional benefits of these exercises include better posture, improved breathing, increased overall strength and mobility, decreased stress response, and enhanced quality of life.

Although the exercises and methods contained in this book are designed to safely address many different causes of back pain, it's still important that you consult your doctor for approval before doing this or any exercise program. If you experience an increase in pain or any cautionary sensations while practicing these exercises, stop immediately and seek the advice of a health-care professional. Even though practicing the exercises in this book may help you avoid extreme medical interventions such as surgery and dependence on prescription medication, this book is not a replacement for medical treatment. Readers in extreme pain should see their doctor. Whatever you do, don't let fear of surgery stop you from seeing your doctor. With the American College of Physicians' new guidelines for back pain treatment promoting the use of nondrug measures first, your doctor should be more likely to work with you on noninvasive solutions, like incorporating the exercises in this book into your treatment regimen.

If you're living with back pain, it's time to take your life back. And I'm going to help you do it. Let's get started.

PART ONE

BACK PAIN BASICS

WHEN SOMEONE SUFFERS from serious back pain, they often describe it as their back "going out" on them. Words have power, so when we use the same passive phrasing we'd use to describe an inanimate object, like a burned-out lightbulb or blown fuse, we're conveying a lack of understanding and responsibility for our personal health. That kind of passive attitude and approach can be a major impediment to healing, which is why it's important to arm yourself with the right information and resources in order to be positive and proactive.

Our bodies are amazing vehicles we've been blessed with to navigate our lives, so we have an obligation to care for them. But we can only effectively do that by taking action and educating ourselves about best practices for getting and keeping our backs healthy and pain-free. By reading this book you are well on your way to doing this. Research published in *JAMA: The Journal of the American Medical Association* found that combining education with exercise actually reduced back pain reoccurrence risk by an additional 10 percent versus exercise alone.

The first section of this book sets the foundation by empowering you with the necessary information to be more proactive in your own pain relief and to improve your relationship with your body. In chapter 1, we'll not only explore the reasons *why* our backs hurt but also look at *how* our backs work, and you'll learn practical ways to relieve pain. Chapter 2 is devoted to explaining why exercise works and why practitioners now recommend it over medication and surgery. It also explores how integrating mind-body techniques with exercise helps heal and strengthen the back. So although you may be eager to jump right into the exercises in part 2, it's important to take the time to first assimilate the information in the next two chapters.

CHAPTER 1

Why Your Back Hurts

Not all instances of back pain can be immediately attributed to a specific cause. Quite often, back pain seems to come on suddenly while you're doing something seemingly innocuous that you've done thousands of times before, like tying your shoes, getting out of bed, or picking up a bag.

When we lack a good explanation for the cause of our back pain, we tend to attribute it to having moved wrong. However, a basic understanding of the anatomy and biomechanics of the spine reveals that there are actually very few "wrong" ways for a healthy spine to move. The key is to understand the spine's form and function so you can maintain a full range of pain-free movement. This chapter examines the causes of back pain, including injury, wear and tear, the interactions of emotions and back pain, and more.

The Anatomy of the Spine

The spine, also known as your backbone, is a complex bony structure that houses the spinal cord, which consists of thousands of nerve endings that relay messages between the brain and body. The spine is both strong and flexible, enabling us to move in all directions and planes of motion while still protecting the spinal cord and bearing the weight of the head and torso. It's an impressive collection of 33 bones, 24 of which make up the 7 cervical vertebrae of the neck, 12 thoracic vertebrae of the mid back, and 5 lumbar vertebrae of the lower back, as seen in the illustration. The first 24 vertebrae are considered articulated, which means they are interconnected by facet joints that allow the vertebrae to move against each other. The remaining bones of the spine consist of nine naturally fused vertebrae: five for the sacrum (triangular bone between the hips) and four in the coccyx (tailbone).

The size, form, and function of vertebrae vary in the different sections of the spine. Unlike any other part of the spine, the cervical vertebrae have openings for arteries that carry blood to the brain. The thoracic vertebrae are attached to the ribs, which wrap around and attach to the sternum (chest bone) in the front. In the lower back, the lumbar vertebrae are the largest in the spine because they're responsible for bearing most of the body's weight. Lumbar vertebrae aren't

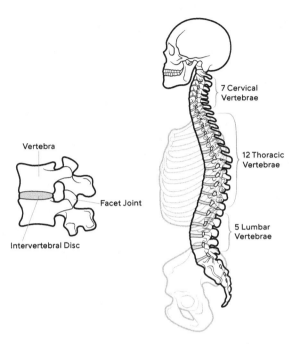

The natural curves of the spine are designed to help create pain-free body posture. Cushioning discs are found between each spinal segment or vertebra.

Labels in figure:
- Vertebra
- Facet Joint
- Intervertebral Disc
- 7 Cervical Vertebrae
- 12 Thoracic Vertebrae
- 5 Lumbar Vertebrae

like the mid back and hips, to take rotational stress off the lower back.

Many people confuse vertebrae with discs, using the terms synonymously. But the two structures are very different. The spine contains 23 discs—one between each of the 24 articulated vertebrae. They're identified according to their position between vertebrae, for example, disc L4/L5. Disc construction is somewhat like a jelly donut, made from soft cartilage with a tougher outside and squishy inside. The water-based contents of the discs are designed to act as shock absorbers and aid vertebral mobility. Consequently, discs must be well hydrated to maintain optimal function. When we're born, our discs are 80 percent water, but, as part of the natural aging process, they dehydrate and get stiffer, making them less able to facilitate movement. When talking about back pain, we hear a lot about discs because, when they're damaged, they understandably lead to pain.

We also have ligaments of dense connective tissue surrounding the spine that keep the column of vertebrae in place while allowing it the flexibility to bend and twist. If the

designed for rotation, like the other parts of the spine; instead, they favor flexion (forward bending) and extension (backward bending). Because of the limitation in lower-back rotation, this is an area where most people tend to actually move "wrong." I'll address this in more depth in chapter 4 as you learn exercises to increase mobility in other areas,

spinal ligaments get overstretched, torn, or wrongly positioned, they decrease the spine's stability, increasing injury risk and causing pain and discomfort.

The spine is naturally curved for optimum stability, mobility, and balance during activity. The cervical and lumbar spine segments are lordotic (curved backward) while the thoracic spine is kyphotic (curved forward). The spine's shape is often described as a soft "S." Although there can be natural genetic variation in the size of the curves in different people, excessive or lack of curvature can cause serious problems.

Muscles That Support and Move Your Spine

When we talk about our back, we are usually referring to the entire muscular structure, not just the bones of our spine. The spine couldn't hold its position or move without muscular support and effort. In fact, without muscles, the spine would be like an unsteady, unsupported tower of blocks. It's therefore important to gain a working understanding of some of your primary back muscles so you can best leverage the exercises in this book to strengthen and restore their ability to support your spine. But don't get hung up on memorizing muscle names. This section is intended to give you an overview of the anatomy and biomechanics of your back, not overwhelm you with information. When these muscles are referenced later in the exercise chapters, you can simply refer back to this section for a reminder of their location and function, if you need to.

To hold us upright and allow movement in all directions, we have sets of paired muscles on either side of the spine in the front, back, and sides of the body. Although these muscles work together in most movements, they can be classified as having primary roles in certain types of movement: extension (backward bending), flexion (forward bending), rotation (twisting), and lateral movement (side bending).

Extensor muscles attach to the back of the spine, and although they're involved in most movement of the back, they are primarily responsible for upright posture and the ability to arch or extend backward. Extensor muscles include the large paired muscles in the lower back and trunk, like the erector spinae, quadrates lumborum (aka the "QL"), and gluteal muscles (glutes). If you suffer from low back pain, you may have heard of one or more of these muscles because they can all impact your low back when strained, tight, or not working properly.

Flexor muscles, often called "hip flexors," attach to the front of the spine to enable activities involving forward bending; the most significant muscle, relative to back pain, is arguably the psoas major, which will be discussed in more detail in the next section.

The paired muscles primarily responsible for rotating and side bending are the obliques, which are generally considered side-waist muscles. They attach to the sides of the spine for twisting, bending, and maintaining posture.

But that's not all. There's one more muscle that influences the spine but is seldom discussed relative to back pain because it isn't one of the paired muscles. It is attached to the front of your lumbar spine and is involved in one of the most vital movement patterns that we make up to 24,000 times a day. The muscle in question is the diaphragm, and the movement pattern is breathing. Let's go over how breathing affects the health of your back.

How Breathing Impacts Your Back

As you can tell by looking at any skeleton, our rib cage is attached to the thoracic spine. Because of this, we can easily understand how our rib cage could impact our spine's position and movement and vice versa. But what most people don't realize is that the diaphragm, our primary breathing muscle, also influences our back in substantial ways because it attaches to both the rib cage and the lower back, making it a significant postural muscle as well as a respiratory muscle.

As the illustration shows, the dome-shaped diaphragm attaches inside the rib cage and has two long tendinous structures, called crura, which attach to the front of the lumbar vertebrae. It's worth noting that the crura are asymmetrical and that the diaphragm's attachment to the lower back overlaps with and runs through the psoas major, our largest, deepest hip-flexing core

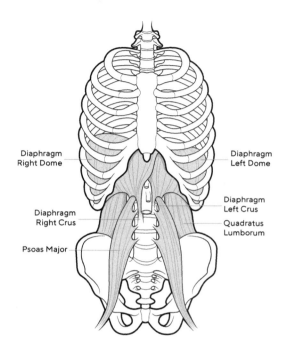

This illustration shows the integrated nature of the spine, rib cage, diaphragm, and primary hip and back muscles.

Diaphragm Right Dome

Diaphragm Left Dome

Diaphragm Left Crus

Diaphragm Right Crus

Quadratus Lumborum

Psoas Major

muscle—and the only muscle in our body that attaches our spine to our legs. This will all come into play later as I introduce you to specific pain-relieving exercises in part 2.

For now, let's focus on understanding the reciprocal relationship between breathing and posture. In the simplest terms, if your posture is bad, your breathing will be bad, and if your breathing is poor, your posture will be poor. That's because how efficiently the diaphragm functions for breathing dictates the position of the rib cage and spine, and the rib cage and spine position affect the ability of the diaphragm to function. Unfortunately, due to chronic stress, illness, injury, sedentary lifestyle, and other factors, many people develop poor posture and a faulty breathing pattern that is chest oriented and shallow.

Take a breath. Do you feel your shoulders lift more than your lower ribs move? If so, you've likely created a common compensatory means of breathing by lifting your rib cage with your shoulder, chest, neck, and upper back muscles, instead of using your diaphragm. Because we take as many as 1,000 breaths an hour, this compensatory breathing pattern is constantly firing those muscles, causing upper-body tension that locks you into poor posture with your rib cage lifted and flared, shoulders slumped forward, and mid back flattened. And this poor posture leads to chronic low-back tension, a decreased ability to move, and an increased injury risk.

Common Causes of Back Pain

According to the American Chiropractic Association, as many as 31 million Americans suffer from low back pain at any given time. Most of this pain originates in the low back and is from degeneration, muscular stress, mental stress, or a combination of these issues. Here are the most common conditions that result in back pain and the reasons why the pain can manifest.

Age-Related Degeneration

After the age of 30, bone density and muscle mass begin to decrease, as does the health of the spinal discs, which dehydrate and stiffen, becoming less able to cushion the vertebrae. The body's defensive response to degenerative changes in the spine is often to grow new bone and thicken ligaments for support. But thickened ligaments and bone spurs can narrow the space around the spinal cord, leading to spinal stenosis. Without adequate space, the spinal cord is restricted and nerves become irritated. Depending on the location of the stenosis—usually the low back—symptoms include numbness, weakness, or muscle cramps in the back, buttocks, arms, or legs.

Degenerative breakdown can also lead to spinal osteoarthritis, the most common cause of back pain in people over 50. It happens when cartilage and facets of the spine break down, causing stiffness, aching, and weakness, as well as numbness in the arms and legs if nerves are affected by the degeneration.

Spondylolisthesis is a condition in which one vertebra moves forward over the vertebra below it. The vertebral misalignment puts pressure on nerves, which causes pain and can lead to weakness and tingling in the legs. Because of the instability and movement of the vertebrae with this condition, symptoms often come and go suddenly, sometimes shifting from one side of the body to the other.

With all degenerative issues, muscular pain can also be present as muscles defensively tighten and stiffen around areas of degeneration in order to protect the spine.

Physical Trauma

Cases of a "broken back" are rare but vertebral fractures can happen, usually due to severe trauma from a bad fall, sports incident, or automobile accident. But fractures can also happen due to compression, which is generally associated with osteoporosis and degeneration. Women are twice as likely to suffer from a compression fracture as men. Fractures may result in sudden severe back pain or, if they don't impact a nerve, no pain at all.

Disc herniation—when the shock-absorbing discs tear or are pushed out of place between vertebrae—is also common due to accidents or putting a significant physical demand on the spine through lifting, pushing, pulling, or twisting. It can also occur during less extreme movements when instability is already present due to tight hips, degeneration, or poor posture. In those cases, you can herniate a disc simply by putting pressure on your low back when getting out of the car, swinging a golf club, or even just bending over to pet your dog. Pain from disc herniation may be felt at the site of the herniation as well as down other parts of the back and legs if the disc or its leaking contents is irritating a nerve.

Tight Hips/Hip Problems

As covered previously, our low back is not designed for twisting. But when our hips are tight, we have a tendency to put pressure on our low back during twisting movements. Over time, that can compress and break down spinal discs, causing pain and increasing risk of injury. As a defensive measure, low-back muscles will also tighten, causing muscle pain.

Another common hip-related cause of back pain comes from the sacroiliac (SI) joints, which connect the pelvis and hips to the sacrum. The SI joints are involved in carrying the weight of the upper body. When hip and pelvis muscles are tight and put pressure on the SI joints, or the joints themselves become too lax due to degeneration, they can become inflamed, causing pain in the low back and legs.

Piriformis syndrome is a pain in the butt—literally—but can also cause back pain and sciatica, which is nerve pain felt down the back of the legs. The piriformis muscle

BREAK BAD BACK HABITS

Old habits die hard. It may be a cliché, but it's true. And many of those old habits will bring back your former pain. Here are five ways to break bad back habits and continue your progress toward healthier, happier living.

>> Stop slumping

Remember that posture and breathing are intimately connected. Don't just throw your shoulders back when you catch yourself sitting in a slump. Regularly practice the seated posture and breathing exercise from this book to cultivate and maintain good posture—and avoid unnecessary back pain!

>> Switch sides

Yes, human bodies are asymmetrical. But when we overuse our dominant side, we create muscle patterns of weakness and tension, increasing pain and injury. My most successful—and least injured—professional athlete clients are ambidextrous in some manner (for example, playing golf left handed but hitting baseballs right handed). So notice if you are always leaning your weight more to one side. Don't always sit on the same side of the couch. Switch shoulders when you carry your computer bag. Try using your opposite hand for basic activities such as opening doors.

>> Move more

Our bodies need adequate movement throughout the day to keep joints mobile and blood circulating through our muscles, which is why it's important to make opportunities to move more. You might have heard this before, but, if the weather is good, don't hunt for the closest parking spot at the grocery store. And when you have the option of an elevator for one or two flights of stairs, take the stairs. When you need to talk with a friend or colleague, have a walking meeting.

>> Be present

A 2010 Harvard study found that, at any given moment, nearly 50 percent of people are not thinking about their task at hand, leaving them stressed and depressed. And as noted above, both stress and depression are linked to back pain. Conversely, being present in the moment reduces physical and mental stress. Because breathing is our most profound connection to the present moment, using the daily "breathing break" exercises in this book will connect you to the present and reduce the physical and mental stress that can lead to back pain.

>> Take care

The primary goal of this book is to empower you with information and tools to take responsibility for your own self-care. If your back hurts at the end of the day, don't just decide it was a "bad" day. Ask yourself if you practiced all the activities that you know help you avoid the stress and tension that cause you discomfort. After reading this book, you will have learned ways to prevent and alleviate pain, so take action.

stabilizes the hip joint. It's located deep in the buttock area, connecting the spine to the thighbone. If this muscle becomes overly tight, it can compress the sciatic nerve.

Poor Posture/Breathing

Poor posture is any posture that forces the spine out of its natural curves, changing the soft "S" spinal curve to more of a "C." This results in chronically tight and overstretched muscles, tendons, and ligaments holding the spine in an unnatural position. Due to the relationship between breathing and posture, poor posture causes poor breathing with a tight diaphragm that pulls on the lumbar spine. Pain caused by poor posture and breathing tends to be chronic and felt particularly in the upper and lower back where muscles are most impacted by changes to spinal curves.

Sedentary Lifestyle

Our bodies are designed for movement. Spending much of our time sitting causes posture and breathing problems, which, combined with lack of movement, result in stiff, weakened muscles and decreased joint

lubrication, including dehydration of spinal discs. These conditions all contribute to back pain and increased risk of spine injuries and degenerative conditions.

Excess Weight or Pregnancy

Overweight people are at an increased risk for back pain due to the additional pressure on the spine, which can result in herniated discs and pinched nerves. This is especially true for extra weight gain in the belly, such as during pregnancy, that pulls the pelvis forward, compressing the lumbar spine. Additionally, pregnant women can experience back pain related to the production of a hormone that causes joint laxity, intended to help open the hips and pelvis for childbirth. This added laxity can lead to SI joint problems and adversely impact the stability of the spine, particularly if combined with excessive weight gain.

Stress

When under stress, whether from physical or mental issues, our bodies produce a physiological response known as the fight-or-flight response. This puts us into a state of hyperarousal that raises the heart rate and blood pressure and floods the body with stress hormones. It's a survival mechanism, enabling people to react quickly to life-threatening situations. Unfortunately, this response can also kick in due to stressors from the modern world, locking the body in a state of fight or flight that can cause back pain due to chronic muscle tension and hypersensitivity to pain.

Depression

When it comes to back pain, especially long-term pain, there is usually a psychological component. The parts of the brain that perceive pain also regulate mood, which means that pain not only intensifies emotional issues, it can also actually be the cause of depression and anxiety. Research suggests that up to half of the people enduring pain for three months or longer suffer from depression or another mood disorder.

Smoking

If you're a smoker who has back pain, you aren't alone. Smokers are nearly three times more likely to experience low back pain than nonsmokers, because nicotine thickens blood vessel walls, which then restrict blood flow in the lower back. Smoking can increase the likelihood of injury as well as healing time.

Daily Life Takes Its Toll

The ways we position ourselves when we stand, sit, sleep, walk, drive, and do the activities associated with our lifestyle have a significant impact on the health of our backs and our risk of injury. That's why becoming more aware of our backs during daily movements and understanding how we can proactively prevent pain from those movements are essential components of self-care.

Our dominant side plays a significant role in how each of us moves through our daily lives. Although nature designed us to have a dominant side (primarily the right), it can be detrimental to back health when we consistently favor one side. It can be even more problematic if we spend a lot of time at our desk, on our couch, in our car, and so on, because the human body wasn't built for so much sitting.

Think about how you sit in your car or at your desk or even stand at the sink doing dishes. Is your weight centered between your hips or do you tend to lean into your dominant side? Do you hold one shoulder lower (usually on the dominant side) while the other sits higher? Can you see how subconsciously holding that misaligned posture can lead to back pain?

What about the impact of your shoe choice? Or the physical demands of your job? Even how we sleep—position, quality, and amount—factors into back health. Virtually every aspect of daily life influences our ability to prevent back pain. Let's take a look at some aspects where a little education and awareness can go a long way.

Household Chores

Raking leaves and shoveling snow are seasonal chores that often cause back pain, largely due to the fact that we don't do them every day and have a tendency to overdo it when faced with a snow-covered driveway or leaf-filled yard. It's important to be mindful of how you use your body during these chores, switching which side you hold the rake or shovel and taking breaks often. Whenever doing chores that require a twisting motion, like shoveling, raking, or sweeping, focus on twisting from the middle of your back and hips, never your low back. Too many people are told to avoid twisting entirely to avoid back injury, but the truth is that most people just twist incorrectly. The body is designed to rotate quite well from the t-spine (thoracic spine) and hips. It's when people try to rotate from their low back that they hurt themselves. That's why the exercises in this book emphasize stability in the low back and mobility in the thoracic spine and hips.

Everyday chores like rinsing dishes, sweeping the floor, or carrying laundry up the stairs are basic tasks we don't need to give much thought to, so we tend to go through the motions mindlessly. However, did you know that the number-one reason for ER visits is related to falls on stairs? Falls often happen when people are relying solely on muscle memory rather than being present in their activity. It's important to pay attention and be present in your body while performing tasks, particularly if you have back pain or have suffered a previous injury.

The more you are connected to and listening to your body, the less likely you are to move incorrectly or take a wrong step that could result in pain or injury. We'll discuss this more as we look at the importance of the mind-body connection in chapter 2.

Work/Screen Time

Back pain is one of the most common reasons for missing work. And back injuries are the second-most prevalent type of injury to happen at work, according to the Occupational Health and Safety Administration (OHSA). Consequently, back pain is a major reason employees claim workers' compensation. If your job involves heavy lifting, take heed of your back health and safety by employing a good lifting technique that uses your legs and core—not just your back.

Whether you're an office worker, a sports coach, or stay-at-home parent, you probably spend at least part of your day sitting in front of a computer, tablet, or phone screen. When we're sitting, we often lose track of time, forgetting to stand, stretch, and breathe. Setting an alarm to go off at regular intervals can remind you to take a break and move.

Driving and Travel

Thankfully, car seat ergonomics have come a long way over the past decade. That said, prolonged driving is prolonged sitting, which can be tough on your back. Because the pedals and controls are set up to favor the right side, we tend to keep our weight more on that side, which can lead to muscle imbalance and tension. While driving, try to keep your weight evenly distributed in the seat and avoid twisting when getting out of the car, since your back is probably stiffer than normal from sitting. Be sure to take regular breaks to get out of the car to move and stretch.

Sleeping

Everything from how we think and feel to our ability to produce energy and recover from injury is impacted by the quality and quantity of our sleep. If back pain is waking you in the night, there's no way to get the rest you need. Avoid sleeping on your stomach, since it exacerbates stress on your lumbar spine and low-back muscles. Ideally, sleep on your left side. We have a tendency to be pulled more onto the right side of the body due to anatomical asymmetry and cultural right-side dominance, so you want to counter that, if possible. Use a pillow between your knees to facilitate pelvis and spine alignment. If you sleep on your back, use a large pillow under your knees to elevate them and take pressure off your lower back.

Recreation and Sports

If you're a "weekend warrior," you tend to cram all your exercise and recreational activities into the weekend. After five days of being sedentary, it's important to warm your body up and ease into your activity, staying mindful of your limitations, especially if you're over the age of 30. If you are an athlete, no matter how competitive your nature, remember that sports science has, thankfully, helped us evolve past the "no pain, no gain" mentality. Listen to your body so you know when it's telling you to back off versus squeezing that last bit of gas out of your tank.

TRAVEL TIPS FOR BACK PAIN RELIEF

Traveling can be hard on our backs. Being conscientious and proactive is key. For pain-free travel, try these five tips.

>> Stand more

It never ceases to amaze me when everyone sits at the airport gate waiting to get on a plane where they'll inevitably be trapped in their seat for at least an hour and usually much more. Or at rest stops when people sit in their cars checking their phones after a quick trip to the restroom. More studies are showing us the real health dangers of prolonged sitting, but we don't need studies to tell us that it makes our backs hurt! Take advantage of opportunities to stand whenever possible during trips.

>> Breathe better

When we sit for long periods while traveling, our posture begins to suffer, and our breathing follows, creating uncomfortable patterns of muscle tension. Shallow breathing then incites the stress response, increasing physical and mental tension. That's why it's important to take control of your breathing at least once an hour while traveling to restore good posture and prevent stress. Taking just five long, deep breaths once per hour can make a big difference.

>> Stretch out

Traveling means sitting, which means compressed side-waist muscles, overused hip flexors, and tight low-back muscles. If you want to be more comfortable and avoid pain when traveling, you need to stretch out those muscles often. My go-to travel stretch is the Warrior Hip Flexor Stretch (supported version on page 45 and unsupported version on page 117). It helps to do it before, during (if possible), and after travel.

>> Drink enough

This is a mistake too many people make. It's so easy to become dehydrated while traveling. The body is mostly water, and the soft jelly-like material between our spinal segments is primarily fluid. Dehydration decreases joint lubrication and circulation, causing muscle tension and fatigue that exacerbates back pain. It's important to drink enough water but, if possible, drink electrolyte-enriched water, since electrolytes are minerals involved with all cellular processes, including bone and muscle maintenance.

>> Recover, seriously

You might be so relieved to get to your destination that you think just plopping down in a chair or on the bed is all you need to recover from your trip. But it's important to counter the impact of travel in all the ways you can. My favorite post-travel restorative exercise is the Legs Up the Wall (page 39) pose from chapter 3. Simply by taking your legs above your heart you change your relationship with gravity and boost blood flow to refresh and restore your stifled lower body.

CHAPTER 2

The New Exercise Program

Bodies are designed for movement. That's why the latest research on chronic back pain provides increasing evidence that the proactive use of exercise is more effective than commonly prescribed passive measures.

In this chapter, we'll look at the limiting—and even dangerous—impact of traditional treatments and the substantial benefits of exercise over them, especially when you're trying to avoid surgery and return to your normal lifestyle. I'll also share why and how the right kinds of exercise used as self-care are not only healing but also strengthening to both the body and mind in their ability to manage and prevent pain.

The Trouble with Tradition

Back pain is among the top ten reasons people visit the ER and among the top five reasons they see their primary care physicians. Doctors have a lot of experience with diagnosis and treatment of back issues, but some of them are set in their ways, including escalating interventions that too often cause more harm than good.

When you find yourself at the doctor's office due to back pain, you're trying to find out why you are in pain and how to get relief from it. To meet your needs, the conventional approach for most doctors is to order tests and prescribe pain medication. Although this may seem like a logical response, the overuse of methods like MRIs, CT scans, and X-rays as well as narcotic prescriptions can lead to serious problems, including unnecessary surgery, opioid dependency, and even death. A study published in *JAMA: The Journal of the American Medical Association* in 2013 found that the use of CT and MRI scans increased by 57 percent from 1999 to 2010, while narcotic prescriptions rose by 51 percent. Referrals to specialists, including surgeons, increased by more than half.

Unfortunately, there doesn't seem to be any correlation between the increase in testing and pain meds with the reduction of pain and disability. In fact, a review published in *JAMA: The Journal of the American Medical Association* of 20 trials, involving nearly 7,300 patients with chronic back pain, found that narcotic pain medications didn't provide significant relief. What's more, medication side effects caused half of the patients to cease use and drop out of the trial early.

There is, however, a correlation between a rise in advanced imaging tests and back surgery. Because imaging can show herniations, spinal stenosis, arthritis, and other malformations and degenerations, patients who become aware of these issues—regardless of whether their symptoms and pain are commensurate with what the imaging shows—are often led to believe that surgery is the only way to solve them. And this happens regularly in conventional medicine even though the surgery is often treating the symptom rather than the true cause of the pain. As a result, many back pain patients end up having more than one surgery because their symptoms return.

For example, a disc herniation might be visible in an MRI, but if the herniation was caused by a change in the spinal curve due to poor posture habits, it cannot be fixed with surgery since the underlying cause remains untreated, and the patient's poor posture will continue to put pressure on the spine. It's the less-aggressive, exercise-based therapies that have been shown to reduce, and often

alleviate and prevent, symptoms and any further damage. That's because exercises address the common causes of back pain such as muscle issues, posture and breathing problems, and overall lack of healthy movement.

An additional danger of too much testing is that once someone receives a diagnosis and sees an image that identifies their spine as having an issue, they begin to identify with that issue, seeing themselves as permanently broken or damaged, as opposed to experiencing a temporary pain. This can lead to lowered quality of life and even a cycle of increased pain and injury as patients become less and less active out of fear. One look at my Instagram account and you'll see that I'm very active and far from broken, despite the fact that MRIs have shown I have multiple disc herniations in my neck and low back, as well as cervical spinal stenosis and signs of arthritis and degeneration. Admittedly, seeing the images and hearing the diagnosis was startling, but thankfully I am educated about how my spine works, and I know how to get out of and stay out of pain—even with those conditions. If I identified with the

QUESTIONS TO ASK YOUR DOCTOR

Your doctor can take a number of actions to find answers for you. It's important to tell your doctor about your lifestyle and treatment goals (for example, active or sedentary lifestyle, getting out of pain and staying out of pain without narcotic dependence, being able to continue career and recreational activities) during this process. Ask the following questions to ensure that the steps taken best meet your needs.

If your doctor . . .

>> **Orders an imaging scan (X-ray, MRI, CT scan):**
- What is she or he looking for with imaging?
- What are the risks of not doing imaging tests right away?

>> **Provides a diagnosis:**
- What factors about my condition indicate this diagnosis?
- What does this diagnosis contraindicate?
- What's the prognosis?
- Where can I learn more about it?
- Can I safely practice the self-care exercises in this book?

>> **Prescribes an opioid painkiller:**
- Are there non-narcotic alternatives?
- If prescribed, can she or he require authorization for refills?

>> **Prescribes bed rest:**
- Why is this the best approach?
- How long will I have to stay in bed?
- What is the course of action after rest to prevent future pain and injury?

>> **Suggests surgery:**
- Why does my condition require such an extreme treatment?
- Are there alternative therapies that can be tried first?
- What are the risks?

>> **Refers you to a physical therapist or other alternative therapy specialist:**
- How does this therapy work to alleviate and/or prevent my pain?
- What is a good resource for learning more about this therapy?

MRIs, rather than staying active to correct and counter their impact, I would not be able to do my job or live my active, fulfilling life. That's another reason why I'm writing this book—so I can help you avoid this mistake.

Although the Centers for Disease Control (CDC) recommends that health-care providers prescribe narcotics for pain relief under screened and monitored circumstances *only* after nonopioid treatments are found to be insufficient for pain management, pain pill prescriptions are usually a traditional physician's first course of action. That was the case with my first bout with back pain, and I'm willing to bet that the majority of the 80 percent of the population with back pain have had narcotic prescriptions in their medicine cabinets, too.

The fact is that over-the-counter anti-inflammatory analgesics can provide more relief with fewer side effects and serious risks than opioids. The risk of addiction and overdose increases dramatically the longer you take opioids. And, as we know, most back pain is a chronic condition, so without adequate treatment the need for pain relief rarely abates for long. According to the CDC, overdose deaths involving opioid pain relievers continue to rise, exceeding deaths involving heroin and cocaine combined.

Clearly, traditional treatment can come with serious risks. But we can avoid those risks by educating and empowering ourselves to be progressive and proactive in the management of our back pain, using non-narcotic, noninvasive treatment whenever possible.

Exercise as Self-Care

Our bodies are our responsibilities. Unless we're severely disabled and must rely on care from others, it's up to us to ensure that our bodies function well enough to live a happy, healthy life. In a recent *Consumer Reports* survey of people with back pain, one in four respondents stated that a back pain episode had "severely" interfered with the physical and emotional quality of their lives.

It's difficult to live happily while in pain. It can make us feel powerless. But the ability to exercise gives us back our power. And the right kinds of exercise can give us control over not only the pain, but also many facets of our well-being. It's widely known that exercise has numerous benefits for your mind and body, from enhancing your mood to increasing your strength. Studies abound showing the positive impact of exercise on many debilitating conditions, including back pain. In 2016, *JAMA: The Journal of the American Medical Association* released a report based on a sweeping review of 21 studies on back pain, covering treatment methods for more than 30,000 participants. The report's authors found that the proactive use of exercise was more effective at treating and preventing back pain than commonly prescribed passive methods like support belts, orthotics, and rest.

Unlike pain medication and, in some instances, surgery, exercise doesn't simply address the symptoms to get you out of pain for the short term; it works for the long term. As mentioned previously, exercise works because it can treat the most common causes of back pain, and when done correctly, it increases your ability to prevent pain flare-ups. Because muscular issues cause most back pain, strengthening and mobilizing the muscles that support and move

the spine will reduce and prevent pain by enabling your body to move optimally.

Once you're empowered with the right exercises and you begin experiencing their benefits, you'll find that you're more and more motivated to exercise. That's because bodies are designed to reward us for giving them what they need to be healthy and strong. Exercise impacts our physiology, increasing feel-good hormone production and decreasing our stress response. And just like anything that feels good and produces positive results, you'll want more of it.

With the American College of Physicians now promoting guidelines for back pain treatment that favor exercise-based measures first, more doctors specializing in back pain are integrating exercise therapies into their protocols, even adding yoga and Pilates instructors to their practices. The *Consumer Reports* survey found that over 80 percent of back pain sufferers surveyed who had tried yoga and other mind-body exercises reported that it helped them.

Let's go back to those answers we're seeking when we go see the doctor for back pain. We desperately want to know why we're in pain and how to get out of it. In our desperation, we often settle for any traditional means of relief, even if it's temporary. Wouldn't it be great if, instead of being shown imaging that make us feel broken and being prescribed narcotics that leave us feeling out of control, doctors reassured us that we have the power to not only get out of pain but also to move better and feel better than we did before our back pain started? That's what exercise-based self-care can do for us.

Making the Mind-Body Connection

What is the mind-body connection?

On the most basic level, it's the connection between mental and physical health. I like to describe it as the bridge that enables the brain and body to act as a whole, complete unit. It's a brilliant aspect of human design. When it's functioning well, it serves to conduct a beautiful orchestra that restores and sustains us. But when it's disconnected, it wreaks havoc on our well-being.

Mind-body practices, like yoga, tai chi, and mindfulness meditation, are intended to train your mind-body connection, increasing awareness of both your physicality and your ability to be present within your body. By cultivating that connection, you're fostering a sense of self-love and honor for your body while honing your ability to respond to its needs. Doesn't that sound like a more desirable and sustainable means of managing your back health? Rather than waging war against your pain—furthering the disconnection of your mind and body and, unknowingly, battling yourself—you have the power to heal yourself.

I realize that it may sound a little "out there" for some people. I understand. Remember, I work with pro athletes, some of whom have spent their entire lives viewing their body solely as a machine. It's almost as though they see their bodies like a race car, where they're merely a driver relying on the pit crew for management. But even for professional drivers, there can be no point where the car ends and the driver begins when you're traveling at speeds in excess of 200 mph. You may not be a race car driver, and your body may not be a streamlined sports car. But it's the vehicle you've been

LISTEN TO YOUR BODY

Overreacting to pain and passively putting its treatment into someone else's hands can lead to unnecessary tests, medications, and procedures that slow your recovery and create other issues.

The more in tune you are with your body, the more you can differentiate between cautionary sensations that signal you to avoid a particular movement or position and less severe sensations such as muscle tension and joint stiffness that you should work through for recovery. It also helps you recognize when you're feeding into dominant-side tendencies that put too much emphasis on one side of the body. That kind of awareness will empower you to make your own adjustments during exercise, as well as in the daily movements of your life, to create more ease and comfort.

You'll find that the exercises in this book are designed to foster your ability to listen to your body. This will help you create a powerful mind-body connection that will not only help you avoid being over-reactive to pain and become more responsive to the sensations you feel, but also serve as a motivating force in your own self-care.

blessed with to navigate your life. How well you coalesce with the driver's seat will be a major determining factor in the quality of your life.

The primary aspect of your mind-body connection that "powers" your vehicle is your autonomic nervous system (ANS), specifically two parts of it:

SYMPATHETIC
"Fight or Flight"
High-alert, reactionary state
Increased blood pressure
Increased heart rate
Increased stress response

PARASYMPATHETIC
"Rest and Repose"
Down-regulated, restful state
Decreased blood pressure
Decreased heart rate
Decreased stress response

When these two parts are in balance, their mechanisms save us and restore us in perfect sync. Since the dawn of time, "fight or flight" has helped people survive, and "rest and repose" has helped people fall asleep at night. Beyond that, by dictating which chemicals are sent to the brain, they influence every aspect of how we think and feel, so homeostasis of the ANS is critical to our well-being. When the ANS is askew, so is the function of the body and mind. Whether due to the stressful demands of a career, surviving a traumatic event, or dealing with constant back pain, the ANS can get thrown off and hold us more in a state of fight or flight. For back pain sufferers, this exacerbates pain by heightening the pain response and hindering the ability to recover.

A major characteristic of the stress response to pain is shallow, rapid breathing. Combine that with the poor posture of most screen-addicted Americans, and chances are they've fallen into the habit of breathing high in the chest rather than deeply in the lungs. As I explained previously, that causes a cascade of pain-inducing muscular issues.

Even without a stressor present, rapid, chest-oriented breathing caused by bad posture can actually initiate the sympathetic fight-or-flight aspect of our nervous system. The result is a vicious cycle, locking you in a chronic, debilitating physiological state. But, with a stressor like back pain present, fight-or-flight turns on, quickening breathing and increasing heart rate, blood pressure, and stress hormone production.

All of that said, if the ANS is the engine of the mind-body connection, then breathing is the key to access it. Breathing is the only facet of the autonomic nervous system we can control. We can leverage that control to dictate which aspect of the ANS is switched on at any given point.

We know that our sympathetic fight-or-flight response creates shallow, rapid breathing. But did you know that we can also use breathing to stimulate a parasympathetic response? In as little as 90 seconds of functional deep breathing, you can elicit a relaxation response that lowers blood pressure, heart rate, and stress hormone levels. That's why breathing exercises are a major component of all mind-body practices. And it's why breathing instruction is included with all the exercises in this book. Breathing is not just the key to unlocking your mind-body connection, it's a superpower for overcoming stress and living a healthy, happy, pain-free life.

Let's get started on the exercise program so you can see for yourself!

PART TWO

THE EXERCISES

NOW THAT YOU'RE empowered with the right information about your back pain, it's time to start your exercise program!

The exercises in this section are broken down into three chapters:

Chapter 3: Exercises to Relieve Pain
Chapter 4: Exercises to Regain Strength and Mobility
Chapter 5: Exercises for Maintenance and Prevention

The first step to healing your back is getting you out of pain. The exercises in chapter 3 are designed to do just that. For the most part, these are more stretching and restorative postures rather than corrective exercises. Even though a few of them are repeated in the maintenance exercises in chapter 5, they are primarily designed to alleviate your pain in the short term so you're better prepared to put in the effort to regain your strength and mobility for pain-free movement over the long term.

Although stretching can feel really good, it's important to understand that it's only ever a temporary solution on its own. When pain is present, muscles are tightening because they're either being overused to compensate for an issue with another muscle, like lack of proper firing, or to protect an area because there's an injury or damage. Consequently, you can't simply stretch away back issues without incorporating corrective exercises. Over time, too much stretching will cause instability that could lead to greater injury.

I've broken the exercises in chapters 3 and 4 into phases to gradually move you away from a sole focus on the areas of tension into a more integrated approach that emphasizes strengthening movement through a full range of motion, in addition to stretching.

In chapter 4, I address that range with exercises to enhance stability and mobility of the spine through all of its functional movements: flexion (forward bending), extension (backward bending), lateral movement (side bending), and rotation (twisting). The exercises are also designed to restore strength, alignment, and function of the primary supporting areas of the body like the pelvis/hips, rib cage, and core muscles, especially the diaphragm and psoas, whose importance was discussed in part 1. Phase 2 exercises are intended to progress you into greater strength in an enhanced range of motion.

Chapter 5 is all about maintenance and prevention. Most of the exercises in this chapter are repeats of exercises from previous chapters that you'll have already mastered and can do easily and regularly. By doing them several times a week—if not daily—you will continue to reinforce the healthy movement you've achieved that keeps you out of pain. And because you'll also have established a strong mind-body connection, you'll be more aware of when you need to do the exercises, or if you need to go back and use exercises from chapters 3 or 4 to relieve pain or regain strength.

In addition to the exercises in this book, there are a number of alternative therapies you can incorporate into your self-care program. In chapter 6, I outline some of the most common therapies and explain their pros and cons. I recommend taking a look at them to determine whether any might be appropriate for you and finding out if your insurance will cover them. I'm definitely not suggesting you use any of these therapies *instead* of the exercise program in this book, but I do encourage you to consider the possibility of using them *in addition* to it. Personally, both massage and acupuncture were helpful in alleviating my pain after my second back injury. In addition, foam rolling, a self-myofascial release (SMR) technique I explain in chapter 6, is a regular part of my own self-care maintenance program.

You'll notice that at the end of every exercise chapter, I've included exclusively mind-body exercises such as mindfulness meditations and relaxation techniques. But don't consider them afterthoughts just because they are at the end! They're primary components of your program that you'll find highly effective. Once you reach the maintenance stage, you can use any or all of these exercises as needed. I highly recommend a daily mindfulness meditation practice in addition to the "10-breath breaks" you'll have been doing consistently throughout chapters 3 and 4.

At the beginning of each chapter and within each exercise's instructions, I let you know how to do the exercises and at what point to progress to the next phase. I also provide insight for determining which exercises are most appropriate for you. As you advance through the program, decreasing your pain and increasing your body awareness, you will be empowered to select the exercises that work best for you.

Remember that every exercise should be approached as a tool for not only enhancing your back health but also your mind-body connection. As such, use these exercises as opportunities to train yourself to treat your body with respect and kindness. Do not force yourself into positions or approach the exercises with anything other than a sense of self-care. While practicing the exercises, focus on noticing all the sensations you experience while maintaining the ability to breathe deeply. If at any point it becomes difficult to take a deep breath, back off until you can breathe well again.

To practice the exercises, you'll need:

- A yoga or exercise mat
- A foam yoga block
- A couple of towels, thin pillows, or foam pads
- A large pillow or bolster
- A chair that allows you to sit comfortably with your feet on the floor and knees at a 90-degree angle

Important Note

Stop doing any exercises that increase your pain or simply feel "wrong." As noted in part 1, not all back pain has the same cause or will respond to the same remedy, so not all exercises will work for everyone. The exercises included in this book are designed to address the most common potential causes of back pain. Work with your doctor or other health-care professional to understand the source of your back pain and any associated contraindications, and be sure to get their approval before beginning this or any exercise program.

CHAPTER 3

Exercises to Relieve Pain

et's start on the road to recovery by getting you out of pain.

Try all six exercises in phase 1 to see what works for you. Unless you experience increased pain with a particular exercise, practice all of them daily, along with one or more of the mind-body exercises, for the first five days. After five days, if your pain has decreased, progress to phase 2, replacing the previous exercises with the next six, doing them daily, as well as a mind-body exercise, for another five days. The five-day time frame is only an estimate; it may take a week or more before you're ready to progress.

Listen to your body. Stop immediately and skip any exercises that increase your pain or feel cautionary. And feel free to continue doing any exercises from phase 1 during phase 2, if you feel they work better for you. Once you feel confident in the exercises, and you are experiencing less pain and more ease, you can move on to regaining strength and mobility with the exercises in chapter 4. You decide when you are ready to move on. This is your program—for your back.

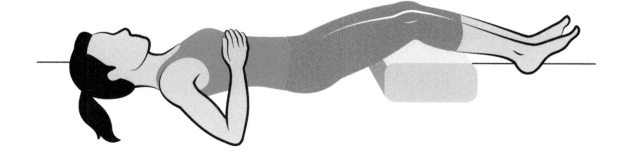

>> **Mind-Body Tip:** As you breathe deeply, focus completely on the sensations you feel, from the air passing through your nostrils to the expansion and contraction of your ribs.

Diaphragmatic Breathing with Legs Elevated

Learning to breathe optimally is the foundation of this exercise program, and it is especially important for this initial phase for pain relief. This is because diaphragmatic breathing can quell the stress response, decrease the reaction to pain, and facilitate the "rest and recover" parasympathetic response. This exercise introduces you to proper rib mechanics for initiating true diaphragmatic breathing, so you can begin experiencing its benefits.

1. Lie on a yoga mat or a firm mattress.

2. Place a large pillow or bolster under the backs of your knees with your legs hip-distance apart. Hip-distance apart means that your ankles and knees are in line with your hips.

3. Place a folded towel or thin pillow under your head to keep your neck neutral. Don't use anything too thick that bends your head forward or tucks your chin.

4. Rest your hands on your lower ribs, where your rib cage splits below your sternum. Focus your attention on how your ribs move as you breathe. During inhalation, your lower ribs should externally rotate (open out) and expand to the sides to accommodate your inflating lungs as your diaphragm flattens and contracts downward. When exhaling, your lower ribs should internally rotate (close in), creating the necessary space for your diaphragm to relax and dome inside your rib cage. With your hands on your ribs, you should be able to "ride" that movement in and out with your breathing.

5. Once you've established the movement of your ribs with inhalations and exhalations, take 5 long, deep breaths at a 5-count inhale, 7-count exhale. Rest for a moment, letting your breathing return to normal (hopefully, it will feel like a "new normal" that's longer and deeper). Repeat for another set of 5 breaths, lengthening your breathing pattern to a 7-count inhale, 9-count exhale, if possible.

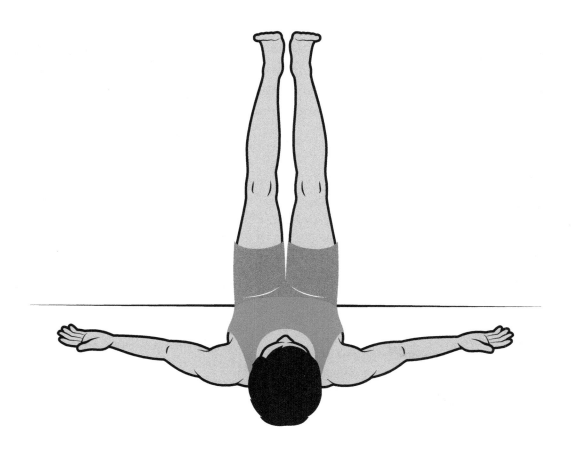

>> **Mind-Body Tip:** Notice the release of tension in your legs and back as gravity allows the weight of your body to settle below them.

Legs Up the Wall

Legs Up the Wall is arguably the most popular restorative yoga pose. It's definitely my favorite! By changing the relationship with gravity and raising the legs above the heart, we promote venous blood flow that eases tension and reduces swelling in the lower body. Additionally, putting the legs straight up stretches the hamstrings (backs of upper legs) to reduce tension on the pelvis and, subsequently, the low back.

1. Sit on the floor with your right shoulder and right hip a few inches from the wall.

2. Lower your left shoulder toward the floor and gently swing your legs straight up the wall with your back and head resting on the ground.

3. If having your legs straight up is too much for you, modify by moving farther away from the wall or resting your legs on a chair seat with your knees bent.

4. If you experience discomfort in your neck or back, place a thin pillow or folded blanket behind your head and/or hips.

5. Remain in this posture for 10 long, deep breaths—or longer, if you find it particularly effective. Because this is a favorite of mine, I usually spend 2 to 5 minutes in it.

6. If you'd like, you can combine this posture with the first exercise, incorporating the "rib riding" breathing.

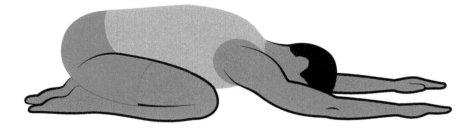

>> **Cautions:** If you have knee issues, be careful because deep knee bending is required for this posture.

>> **Mind-Body Tip:** Focus your attention on allowing all of your back muscles to relax and release into the stretch.

Child's Pose

This is another popular restorative yoga pose. It's especially popular with people with low back pain because of its emphasis on lengthening the lumbar spine. Although it mostly stretches the low back, Child's Pose has a lengthening effect on the entire spine, stretching all the major supporting muscles of the back.

1. Get on your hands and knees on a slightly padded surface, like a yoga mat or carpet. Add extra padding under your knees, if necessary.

2. Be sure to begin with your hips directly above your knees and feet aligned behind your knees with your toes pointed back.

3. Exhale as you lower your hips back and down toward your heels.

4. Inhale as you walk your hands forward as far as they can go comfortably, staying in line with your shoulders. If you experience shoulder pain, walk your hands back to a position where your shoulders no longer hurt.

5. Exhale as you bring your forehead toward the floor. If the floor is out of comfortable reach of your forehead, use a yoga block or pillow as a prop.

6. Take 5 long, deep breaths while you maintain the pose, focusing on letting your hips sink back toward your heels and your back release into the stretch. Come back to all fours for a breath or two and then push your hips back to repeat for another 5 breaths.

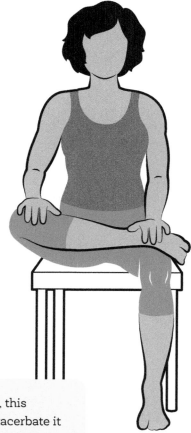

>> **Cautions:** If you have sciatica, this exercise can either soothe or exacerbate it depending on nerve and muscle position. Stop immediately if sciatic symptoms increase, and focus instead on the other exercises in this chapter. If your hips are too tight to get your foot up on your thigh without knee pain, don't force it. Practice the other exercises until your hips open up.

>> **Mind-Body Tip:** Try to find ease in this seated posture by concentrating on letting more and more tension release from your hip with each exhale.

Seated Figure-Four Hip Opener

Because tight hips lead to low-back compensation that leads to pain, it helps to open the hip joint, which is what this posture does. It stretches the muscles of the buttocks, including the piriformis, which can sometimes get tight and trap the sciatic nerve (piriformis syndrome), causing back pain.

1. Sit in a chair with a seat height that enables you to have both feet flat on the ground and your knees at a 90-degree angle. Be sure your feet are hip-distance apart.

2. Inhale as you lift your right foot and guide it with your hands to rest on top of your left thigh just above your knee in a figure-four position, with your foot dorsi-flexed (opposite of a ballet point). To avoid putting unnecessary twisting pressure on your knee joint as you bring your foot into place, focus on using movement within your hip rather than your knee.

3. Exhale as you hold your right shin and sit upright.

4. Maintain this position through 5 long, deep breaths. Repeat the same steps with the other leg.

5. For a deeper stretch, as you hold your shin and exhale, lean forward. Make sure to hinge from your hips when you lean. Don't bend from your back.

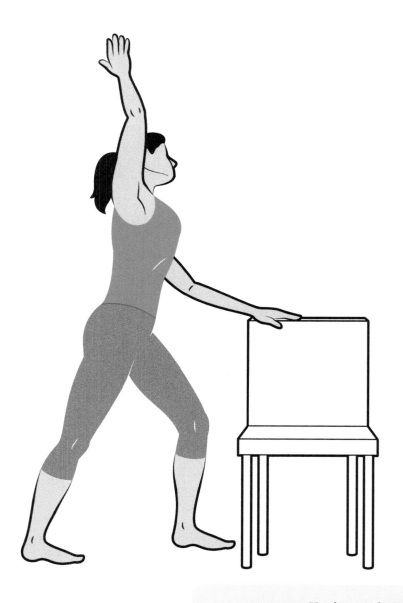

>> **Mind-Body Tip:** You know what your psoas looks like from the illustration in chapter 1, so picture it releasing as you side bend in this posture.

Supported Warrior Hip Flexor Stretch

As you probably are aware, sitting too much contributes to back pain. This exercise releases tension in the areas that get taxed most by sitting: the hip flexors (including the psoas), side-body muscles, and the big paired muscles of the low back.

1. Place your left hand lightly against a wall or chair for support.

2. Step your right foot back into a short lunge, dropping your right heel and pointing your toes out slightly. Bend your left knee to align above your ankle, and keep your back leg straight.

3. Inhale as you lift your right arm up and over your head.

4. Exhale as you side bend to the left. Avoid arching your lower back.

5. As you hold the position, press the front of your right hip forward (like you are trying to tuck your tailbone under you) to release your right hip flexors.

6. Hold for 3 long, deep breaths. Repeat on the other side.

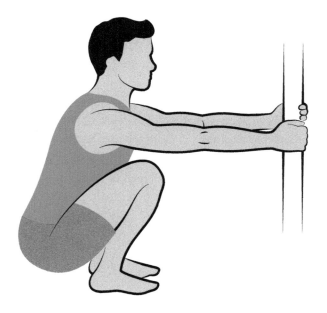

>> **Cautions:** If you have knee issues, be careful because deep knee bending is required for this posture. It's not unusual to feel light-headed upon standing after a round of these. Just continue to hold on to the secure structure and breathe normally until the feeling passes.

>> **Mind-Body Tip:** Use expansive breaths to release your back; with every inhalation, focus on feeling the expansion of your rib cage spreading out and breaking through tension in your back.

Supported Back-Release Squat

This supported squat exercise encourages the pelvis to move into a posterior tilt, which releases low-back extensor muscles on either side of the spine. Like the previous Child's Pose exercise (page 41), it lengthens the spine; however, it does so actively rather than passively because you need to activate deep core and pelvic floor muscles to perform the full squat with proper form.

1. Stand with your feet hip-distance apart and your arms extended forward at shoulder level. Hold on to a pole, door frame, or other secure structure that reaches high enough and low enough to perform the exercise, as shown.

2. Exhale and drop back through your hips and pelvis into a deep squat, walking your hands down the pole as you lower.

3. Maintain weight in your heels with your toes pointed forward. Don't let your feet or knees turn out or heels lift. If you experience discomfort in your ankles, knees, or shins, make sure you're dropping back into your hips as opposed to pushing forward into your knees. You should literally feel like your body weight is hanging off the pole, pushing back into your hips and heels.

4. Take 5 long, deep breaths. Focus inhalations on breathing into your mid back and exhalations on letting your lower back release. Stand and rest a moment, then repeat for another set of 5 breaths.

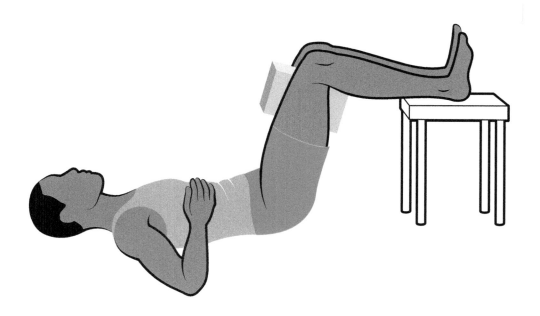

>> **Cautions:** To hold yourself in the bridge position, you should feel the muscular effort in your core and glutes and a little in your hamstrings. You should not feel it in your back. If you do, try setting up again. If you still feel it in your back, skip this exercise.

>> **Mind-Body Tip:** Lifting your hips requires muscular energy. Pay attention to the sensations you feel to distinguish between effort and pain.

Breathing Bridge on Chair

This exercise is the next step in learning to breathe optimally. Unlike the breathing exercise in phase 1, this one requires some effort to activate your glutes (buttock muscles), pelvic floor, and core muscles to hold you in a bridge position. Doing so will strengthen your back by facilitating the proper positioning of your rib cage and the alignment and function of the muscles that support your spine.

1. Lie on your back, knees bent and directly above your hips, and your heels resting on the seat of a chair.

2. Place a foam yoga block, rolled towel, or pillow between your legs.

3. With your arms at your sides, slide your shoulder blades down to relax your upper back and neck. Place a folded towel or thin pillow under your head if needed.

4. Place your hands on your lower ribs, so you can pay attention to and guide the movement of your ribs with your breathing.

5. At the end of an exhale, activate low, deep core muscles and your glutes (buttock muscles) to lift your pelvis a few inches off the floor into a slight bridge.

6. While bridging, inhale through your nose, filling the lowest lobes of your lungs. You should feel your lower ribs externally rotate and expand as opposed to only inflating your upper chest.

7. Exhale, using core muscles to help internally rotate your lower ribs and release your rib cage downward, expelling all air. A complete exhalation is necessary to fully relax your diaphragm.

8. Take 5 long, deep breaths at a 5-count inhale, 7-count exhale while holding your bridge position. At the end of each exhale, pause without taking a breath for a count of 3. The pause should take some effort as you feel your core actively contract, holding your ribs inward without air in your lungs. If you find you can continue exhaling after a 7 count, increase your exhalation time as much as necessary to completely empty your lungs before pausing.

9. After 5 breaths, release from the bridge, rest a moment, then repeat another set.

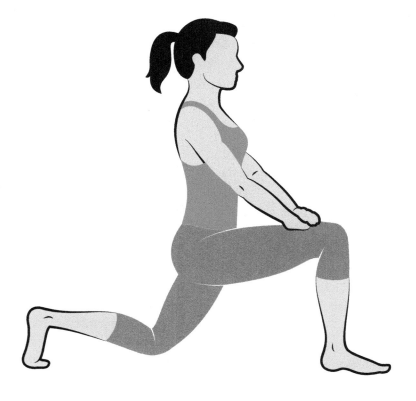

>> **Cautions:** If your low back seems to stay locked on, making it difficult to feel a stretch in your hip flexors, go back to practicing Supported Warrior Hip Flexor Stretch (page 45) as an alternative. Use padding under your knee if you experience discomfort with weight on it against the floor or mat.

>> **Mind-Body Tip:** Remember the connection between the psoas and diaphragm? Use extended exhalations to help lengthen and release your psoas.

Kneeling Lunge

It's important to release tension in the hip flexors, particularly the psoas, which attaches to the lumbar spine. When hip flexors are tight and locked "on," they cause a chain reaction of muscle-firing dysfunction. The glutes oppose the hip flexors and are unable to fire when the hip flexors are locked; to compensate, low-back muscles become overly tight because they turn on to act as hip extensors. This kneeling lunge exercise serves to unravel the dysfunctional chain reaction by stretching the hip flexors while activating the glutes and releasing the low back extensors.

1. Set up in a kneeling lunge position with your right leg in front and left leg behind.

2. Align both feet horizontally with your hips, and position your left knee directly below your left hip and your right knee directly above your right ankle.

3. Place both hands on your right thigh.

4. Inhale as you lengthen your spine to straighten your upper body without arching your back.

5. Exhale to drop the lower ribs in, back, and down while you focus on pressing your left hip forward by tucking your pelvis under.

You should feel your left glute muscles engage to create a stretching sensation in the front of your hip.

6. You may be tempted to push your knee forward to increase the stretching sensation, but that would actually put stress on your low back. Keep your knee aligned above your ankle and focus on the glute firing/hip flexor stretching sensation.

7. Take 3 long, deep breaths in this position. Switch to the other side, with your left leg in front and right leg in back, and repeat the exercise.

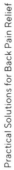

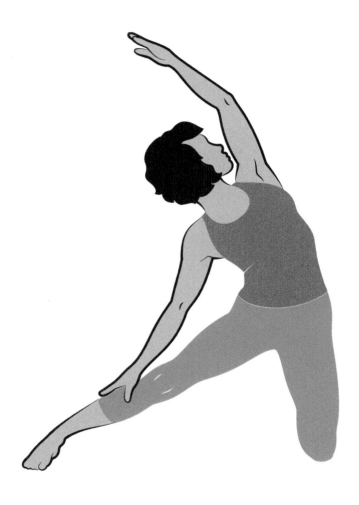

>> **Cautions:** If being on your knees is uncomfortable, use a folded towel or pad under your knees.

>> **Mind-Body Tip:** Stay connected to your breathing in this posture, using your exhales to find ease in the exercise.

Gate Pose

Like the Supported Warrior Hip Flexor Stretch (page 45), Gate Pose moves the spine laterally (sideways), but this exercise enables a deeper side bend, releasing shortened, tense side-waist muscles and the large paired muscles on the sides of your spine, especially the quadratus lumborum.

1. Start in a high kneeling position with your knees hip-distance apart and your hands on your hips.

2. Keeping your left knee directly below your left hip, stretch your right leg out to the right, pressing your foot into the floor with your toes pointing forward.

3. As you inhale, reach your left arm up with the palm facing to the right, and place your right arm on your right thigh.

4. Exhale and side bend to the right, allowing your right arm to slide down your right leg to whatever distance is comfortable.

5. Hold the stretch and take 4 more long, deep breaths for a total of 5 breaths. Focus your breathing on your rib movement to facilitate the stretch. Expand your ribs on the left as you inhale and bring your right ribs in on your exhale.

6. Use an inhalation to lift your torso out of the bend and return to tall kneeling.

7. Rest a moment, then switch legs and repeat all the steps to practice the exercise on the left side.

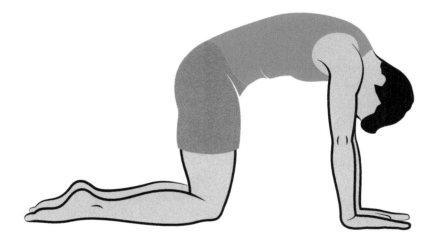

>> **Cautions:** If you've had spinal fusion sur-
gery, parts of your spine may be unable to
move well, so don't force it. If you experience any pain, do not practice this exercise.

>> **Mind-Body Tip:** Visualizing your spine as
a strand of pearls will enable a more precise, fluid movement that avoids hinging
from any one area of your back.

Cat Flow

This is a great exercise for training your mind-body connection by practicing awareness and control of spinal movement. I call it a Cat Flow because the flexion and extension of the spine mimic the movements of an angry cat and a frisky cat.

1. Begin on your hands and knees with your hips stacked directly above your knees, ankles aligned horizontally with your feet, shoulders directly above your wrists, and head neutral, looking at the floor.

2. Inhale and think about your spine like a long strand of pearls that you can articulate, pearl by pearl, starting from your tailbone.

3. Exhale as you tilt your pelvis under to tuck your tailbone to begin taking the shape of a big, angry cat, flexing your entire spine. Create the flexion, segment by segment, stretching your lower back and then continuing to your mid back and, finally, your neck and head. You should feel like your core is engaged and your rib cage is pushed as far back in your body as possible to support the flexion of your spine.

4. As you inhale, start again at your tailbone, tilting it up to gently arch your low back and letting that arch move into your mid back and then to your neck and finally lifting the head to look straight forward. Notice that your head wants to move first, but don't let it. Practice body awareness and control by moving from tailbone to head with full control.

5. Repeat for a total of 5 breaths, exhaling into the rounded-back "angry" cat posture and inhaling into the arched-back "frisky" cat posture.

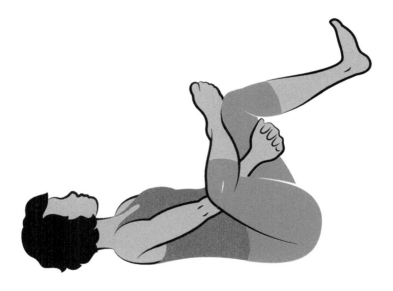

>> **Cautions:** The primary sensation should be a stretch in the outside of your hip; stop if you experience any knee strain or pain.

>> **Mind-Body Tip:** Releasing hip tension should feel good. Allow yourself to tune into the positive sensations of this stretch.

Supine Figure-Four Stretch

Tight hips contribute to low back pain by causing the low back to compensate for lack of hip mobility. And, as discussed in part 1, the lumbar spine is not designed for rotation. This posture will help open your hips.

1. Lie on your back with your knees bent and feet on the floor, hip-distance apart.

2. Bring your right leg up and place your right ankle on your left thigh above your left knee, creating a figure-four position.

3. Lift your left foot to bring your bent left knee toward your left shoulder, keeping it aligned.

4. Reach your hands around either side of your left thigh and clasp your hands together to guide your leg closer to intensify the stretch you feel on the outside of your right hip.

5. As you hold your legs in the stretch, relax your head back to the floor. If it doesn't reach comfortably, put a support under it so your neck can be neutral.

6. Take 5 long deep breaths.

7. Unwind and repeat the stretch on the other side.

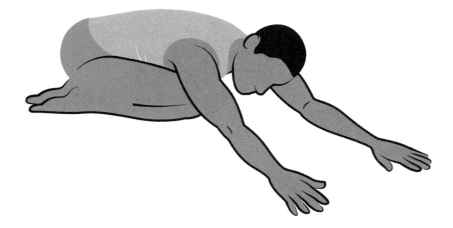

>> **Cautions:** If you have knee issues, be careful because deep knee bending is required for this posture.

>> **Mind-Body Tip:** Notice how the depth of your reach influences the release in each side of your back; move your arms to modulate the sensation to your liking.

Child's Pose with Reach

Child's Pose with Reach lengthens the spine and releases back muscles. Adding the reaching aspect to each side opens up the side body and adds an extra stretch to the muscles along the sides of the low back.

1. On a yoga mat or slightly padded surface, begin on your hands and knees with your hips aligned directly above your knees, ankles aligned horizontally with your feet and toes pointing back, shoulders directly above your wrists, and head neutral. Add extra padding under your knees, if necessary for comfort.

2. Exhale as you lower your hips back and down toward your heels.

3. Inhale as you walk your hands forward as far as they can comfortably go, staying in line with your shoulders. If you experience shoulder pain, back off.

4. Exhale as you bring your forehead toward the floor. If the floor is out of comfortable reach of your forehead, use a yoga block or pillow as a prop.

5. Walk both hands 8 to 12 inches out and over to the right, while keeping your hips back toward your heels and your head centered between your arms.

6. Hold for 5 or more long, deep breaths. Return to the center and hold for another 5 breaths. Repeat on the left side.

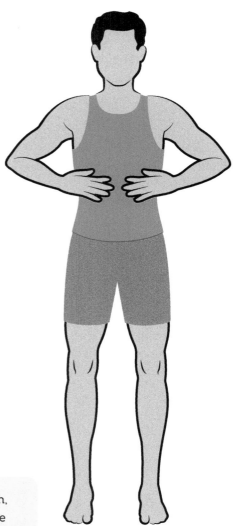

>> **Mind-Body Tip:** After your tenth breath, take an inventory of how you feel. Notice how easily you were able to down regulate (decrease your stress response and feel calm), and use that as motivation to practice this exercise regularly.

10-Breath Breathing Break

As discussed, breathing can help with back pain from both physical and physiological standpoints, since the diaphragm serves as both a postural and respiratory muscle. And in addition to being a direct connection to our autonomic nervous system (see chapter 2), breathing is our most profound connection to the present moment, since it's always happening. By turning your awareness to your breathing, you can cultivate a sense of mindfulness that not only alleviates stress and anxiety but can also make you feel happier.

Better still, we can accomplish these benefits with just a couple minutes of deep, diaphragmatic breathing, initiating your parasympathetic nervous system, which shuts down the stress response by lowering cortisol (stress hormone), blood pressure, and heart rate while increasing oxytocin and endorphins (happy hormones).

1. From any comfortable position—sitting, lying down, or even standing—simply tune into your breathing.

2. Close your eyes or establish a soft focus on a point in front of you.

3. Take conscious control of your breathing, inhaling through your nose and exhaling through your mouth or nose (whichever you prefer). Lengthen and deepen your breath, extending your exhales a bit longer than your inhales, like big sighs of relief.

4. Notice the expansion and contraction of your rib cage and any related sensations you can perceive. Visualize the path of your breath in through your nose, down into your lungs, and back out.

5. If thoughts come into your mind, gently push them aside and maintain your focus on your breathing, as it happens, in the moment.

6. Count 10 breaths like this.

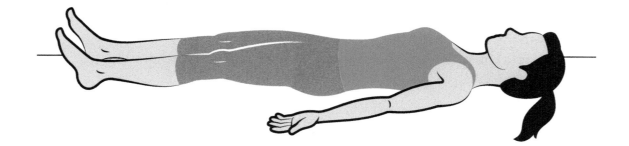

>> **Mind-Body Tip:** As you practice this exercise, tune into the sense of control you establish throughout your body.

Progressive Muscle Relaxation

The goal of this practice is to actively create a sense of relaxation throughout your body by first tensing each area to establish an awareness and connection, and then consciously letting it go. You can do this exercise while sitting, standing, or lying down. I prefer to do it flat on my back with arms and legs slightly open. However, if necessary for comfort, place a rolled or folded towel or pillow under your head, back, or legs.

1. Get into your preferred position with whichever props you may need to feel comfortable.

2. Establish a long, deep diaphragmatic breathing pattern that you can maintain throughout the exercise.

3. On an inhalation, close your eyes tightly while clenching your teeth to tighten your jaw.

4. Exhale to release (but you can keep your eyes gently closed, if you prefer), softening your face, jaw, and tongue.

5. Inhale fully, expanding every part of your rib cage, and hold your breath, creating tension in your chest, upper back, and neck.

6. Exhale to release completely.

7. Inhale and squeeze your hands into fists, tensing all the muscles of your arms.

8. Exhale to release.

9. Inhale to squeeze the muscles of your bottom and pelvic floor while also tightening your abdomen.

10. Exhale to release.

11. Inhale to curl your toes, while trying to activate all the muscles of your legs.

12. Exhale to release.

13. Take 10 or more long, deep breaths while resting in the awareness of a state of complete relaxation. If your mind wanders and you lose track of your count, start over.

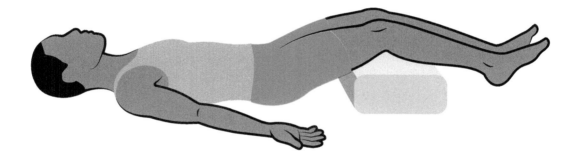

>> **Mind-Body Tip:** Let your senses be completely immersed in the visualization of the numbers, the feeling and sound of your breathing, and the awareness of your body relaxing into your bed.

20-Breath Backward Count for Sleep

Sleep is essential for healing. Your nervous system needs the opportunity to spend time in its "rest and restore" state to facilitate and support the recovery processes of both body and mind. This exercise is kind of like counting sheep . . . but way more effective and beneficial! Pairing deep breathing with backward-counting meditation is a simple yet effective way to focus and relax a wandering mind. And because the diaphragm also works as a postural muscle—attaching to the rib cage and lumbar spine (low back), and running through the hip flexors—diaphragmatic breathing promotes proper rib cage, back, and pelvis position, which decreases the likelihood of waking due to discomfort or the need to change position.

1. Get comfortable in bed with your head on your pillow and another pillow placed under your knees. If you prefer a side-lying position, lie on your left side with a pillow between your legs.

2. Inhale through your nose, filling the lowest lobes of your lungs and back of your rib cage. You should feel your lower ribs expand outward as opposed to only inflating your upper chest. Exhale and focus on your lower ribs internally rotating and descending. It's important that you feel your rib cage release downward as you exhale.

3. Lengthen and deepen your breathing to match this pattern: 5-count inhalation, 7-count exhalation, and 3-count pause after exhalation.

If it's difficult, simply establish a breathing pattern with a longer exhale than inhale and slight pause after exhaling.

4. Once you've established the breathing pattern, begin counting your breaths backward from 20 to 1. Create an image of each number in your mind's eye with each breath. I imagine big, round, white numbers on a light blue background, like fluffy clouds emerging in the sky with each breath I take.

5. If you still haven't drifted off after 20 breaths (about 3 to 4 minutes), repeat the process, starting at 30 or 40. If your mind wanders and you lose track of your count, start over.

CHAPTER 4

Exercises to Regain Strength and Mobility

Congratulations! You have completed the exercises in chapter 3, which means that you're ready to get stronger and move better! Because the following exercises are corrective exercises to address the imbalances and weaknesses that are likely instigating your back pain, it's important that you practice body awareness and use precise alignment.

Follow the directions exactly, ensuring that you properly balance your weight and aren't allowing your center of mass to sit in one hip or leg more than the other, unless the exercise instructs you to do so. Pay attention to your feet and knees, as they serve as windows into hip and pelvis position; if they turn out, it's likely that you're opening your hips or rotating your pelvis.

This chapter introduces twisting exercises that focus on creating healthy spinal rotation in the mid back and neck—never the low back, which isn't designed for rotation. Twisting should always be approached with care. None of these exercises should cause pain, so never force a twist or ignore pain.

As you practice these exercises, decide which ones work for you. Begin by trying

all of the exercises in phase 1. Practice the Breathing Bridge on Chair (page 49) and Seated Posture Exercise with 10-Breath Breathing Break (page 107) daily and then select five additional exercises from the first group to practice every other day for two weeks. You can continue to do any of the pain-relieving exercises from chapter 3 on a daily basis as well. The idea is for you to get to know your body and what it needs, so you decide which exercises feel like they help you the most.

After at least two weeks of phase 1, when you feel ready to progress, begin swapping out your every-other-day exercises for phase 2 options. Within a month or so, you should be able to zero in on the movements that prove most effective for you. Continue doing them three to five times per week as part of your overall physical fitness program, but, once you feel you are completely out of pain and moving optimally, you can transition into more of a maintenance program, as outlined in chapter 5.

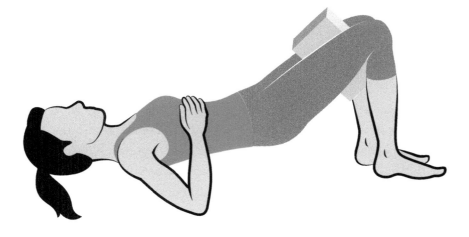

>> **Cautions:** To hold yourself in the bridge position, you should feel the muscular effort in your core and glutes and a little in your hamstrings. You should not feel it in your back. If you do, try setting up again. If you still feel it in your back, skip this exercise or go back to the Breathing Bridge on Chair (page 49) exercise, if that one worked better for you.

>> **Mind-Body Tip:** Pay close attention to the movement of your lower ribs as they expand out when you inhale and move in, back, and down as you exhale.

Breathing Bridge

This is my go-to everyday exercise for strengthening and reinforcing proper breathing biomechanics because it promotes complete core engagement and pelvic/hip alignment to support correct spine position. Breathing Bridge is the starting exercise in all of my clients' programs, and once you master it, it will be a fundamental part of your maintenance program as well.

1. Begin on your back with your knees bent and feet on the floor hip-distance apart, about six inches from your bottom.

2. If necessary, use a folded towel under your head to keep your neck neutral.

3. Place a foam yoga block between your legs to engage the inner thighs and avoid your hips externally rotating and knees splaying out.

4. With your arms at your sides, slide your shoulder blades down to relax your upper back and neck.

5. Place your hands on your lower ribs, so you can pay attention to and guide the movement of your ribs with your breathing.

6. On an exhalation, as you draw your low ribs in and down toward your waist, engage your low, deep core to initiate lifting your hips a few inches off the floor, as you did in Breathing Bridge on Chair (page 49).

7. While bridging, inhale through your nose, filling the lowest lobes of your lungs. You should feel your lower ribs expand outward as opposed to only inflating your upper chest.

8. Exhale, using core muscles to help bring your lower ribs in, and release your rib cage downward, expelling all air. A complete exhalation is necessary to fully relax your diaphragm.

9. Take 5 long, deep breaths at a 5-count inhale, 7-count exhale while holding your bridge. At the end of each exhale, pause without taking a breath for a count of 3. The pause should take effort as you feel your core actively contract, holding your ribs inward without air in your lungs. If you find you can continue exhaling after a 7 count, increase your exhalation time as much as necessary to completely empty your lungs.

10. After 5 breaths, release from the bridge, rest a moment, then repeat for another set.

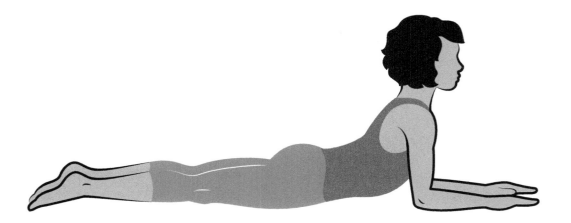

>> **Cautions:** If you have a neck injury or you experience neck pain when doing the head turns, only hold the posture for 3 breaths and don't do the head turning.

>> **Mind-Body Tip:** Be mindful about how you create the arch in your back, actively using muscular support in your mid back—never hinging from your low back.

Sphinx with Head Turns

This exercise promotes mid-back extension while lengthening the low back; it also strengthens the shoulder girdle and opens the front of the shoulders and chest to counter slumped posture. And because the neck is part of the spine, this also addresses cervical rotation.

1. Lie prone (on your belly) resting on your forearms with your elbows directly under your shoulders.

2. Exhale as you press down through your forearms as though you're trying to slide your belly forward through your arms, to create length in your low back. At the same time, move your shoulder blades down toward your waist. This will activate the mid-back muscles essential for thoracic spine extension while inhibiting the muscles of your upper neck and chest that limit mobility.

3. Hold the posture for 3 long, deep breaths.

4. Inhale to turn your head right and exhale back to center; inhale to look left and then exhale back to center.

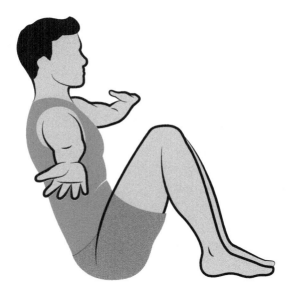

>> **Mind-Body Tip:** Sometimes the mind has difficulty connecting to deep core activation; make it the focus of your attention during this exercise.

Roll-Into-a-Ball Core Exercise

This exercise does double duty by turning off tight, overactive low-back extensor muscles while strengthening the supporting muscles of the groin, pelvic floor, and core. Most people know a strong core is a key component in fighting back pain, but many don't realize that it's important to strengthen firing patterns, not just muscles in isolation. This exercise is effective because it integrates the pelvis and hips.

1. While seated, curl yourself up into a ball with your feet together on the floor, your big toes touching.

2. Keep your knees together to engage the adductors (groin muscles) for hip and pelvic floor stability. If you have difficulty keeping your knees together, modify by separating your feet and squeezing a foam yoga block between your knees.

3. Start with your arms straight out in front of you at shoulder height with your palms pressed together.

4. Inhale as you reach your arms out to the sides, keeping them at shoulder height and rotating the palms up. Don't let your shoulders rise. Use the muscles of your mid back to firmly keep your shoulder blades and shoulders down as you open your arms out.

5. Exhale as you bring your arms together in front of you.

6. Repeat twice more. Drop your knees out to rest, releasing your groin and hips; if hip mobility is limited, additional hip-opening postures are recommended.

7. Repeat for another set of 3.

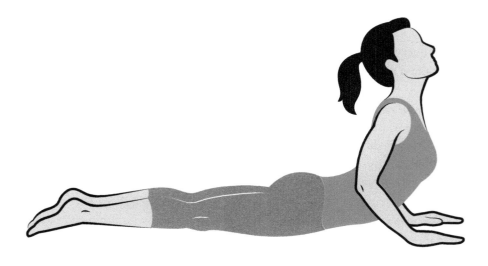

>> **Mind-Body Tip:** Spinal extension (back arching) exercises should only be practiced with mindfulness—and without pain. Use caution and care to create healthy movement.

Cobra

Similar to the Sphinx with Head Turns (page 71) position, this exercise strengthens back muscles and enhances spinal mobility, but it requires greater muscle activation through the mid back—essential posture muscles for helping stabilize your shoulder blades and avoiding a painful slumping posture. Enhancing movement and stability in the shoulder girdle and mid back helps prevent compensations that overwork low back muscles.

1. Lying prone (on your belly), place your palms on either side of the middle of your rib cage, your elbows bent and snug to your sides.

2. Press through your palms as though you're trying to slide your upper body forward through your arms, creating length in your lumbar spine (low back).

3. Inhale as you slowly begin straightening your arms and lifting your shoulders.

4. Exhale and focus on drawing your shoulder blades down toward your waist, feeling your mid-back muscles engage to create and sustain extension in your spine.

5. Take 5 long deep breaths. Rest a moment, then repeat for another set of 5 breaths.

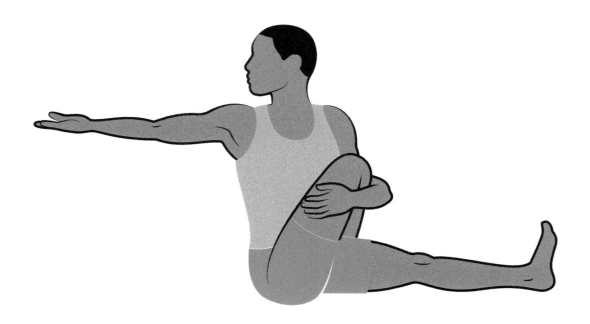

>> **Cautions:** If you have sciatica, this exercise can either soothe or exacerbate it, depending on nerve and muscle position. Stop immediately if sciatic symptoms increase, and focus on the other exercises in this chapter.

>> **Mind-Body Tip:** Remember that healthy spinal twists happen in the mid back; focus your attention on your thoracic spine and rib cage movement.

Seated Bent-Knee Twist

Twisting should always be approached with caution, particularly if you have back pain. This exercise stretches the outside of your hips while also working on twisting from the thoracic spine.

1. Sit with both legs straight out in front of you.

2. Bend your right knee and cross your right foot over your straight left leg. Place your foot on the outside of your left leg and press it into the floor.

3. If your hips are too tight to plant your foot on the outside of your opposite leg without knee pain, don't force it. Modify by placing the foot on the inside of the leg, without crossing over.

4. Wrap your left arm around your right leg as shown in the illustration.

5. Inhale and reach your right arm forward at shoulder height with the palm up.

6. Exhale and rotate from your mid back to the right, moving your right arm behind you and looking back over your shoulder.

7. Hold and take 3 long, deep breaths. Focus the inhalations on expanding your rib cage to the right and exhalations on internally rotating your left lower ribs to help you twist.

8. Remember to keep your straight left leg grounded, with your left foot pointed straight up (not letting your leg rotate outward) and your right foot firmly planted.

9. Release with an exhalation, reverse the legs, and twist to the left for an equal length of time.

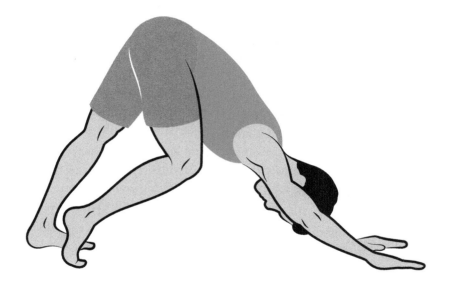

>> **Cautions:** If you can't perform 180 degrees of shoulder flexion (comfortably raising both arms straight above your shoulders), don't force this position. Only go into it as deeply as your shoulders allow.

>> **Mind-Body Tip:** Too often in yoga, we can get hung up on how we think a pose should look. Concentrate on how you feel rather than how you might look.

Bent-Knee Down Dog with Pedal Out

Downward Dog is one of the most recognized traditional yoga postures, but it's not necessarily the easiest. Even this modified version requires total-body effort. But it's worth it because it simultaneously lengthens the spine, strengthens the core and shoulders, and stretches out the backs of the legs—all of which promote a healthy, pain-free back.

1. Start on your hands and knees with your hands slightly forward of your shoulders and your hips directly above your knees.

2. Turn your toes under and exhale as you lift your knees, engaging your quadriceps (muscles of the front of your legs) to begin straightening your legs while bringing your pelvis up and back. Do not fully straighten the legs. Maintain a bend in your knees.

3. Avoid rounding your low back. Your core should be engaged for support while your low back lengthens. The tailbone should serve as the apex of the posture, like an A-frame.

4. Use your mid-back muscles to pull your shoulder blades toward your waist, broadening your upper back and lengthening your spine.

5. Keep both knees bent and take a breath or two as you acquaint yourself with the position, being mindful of all the points of instruction and the corresponding sensations of strengthening and stretching in your body.

6. As you take 5 long, deep breaths, slowly press one heel down, straightening that leg while bending the opposite knee, then switching sides—going back and forth to "pedal" out your heels. This will create a stretch in the back of your legs, especially your calves.

7. Return to your hands and knees, rest a moment, then repeat for another set of 5 breaths or so.

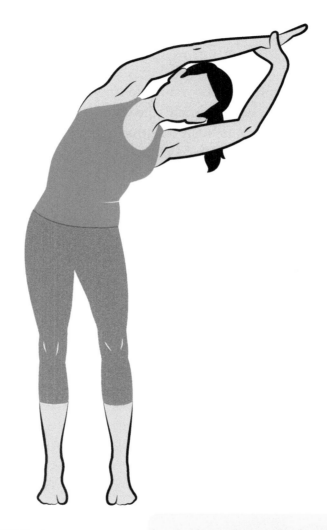

>> **Cautions:** If you have difficulty avoiding an arch in your low back while doing this exercise, continue practicing Gate Pose (page 53) as an alternative until you feel more comfortable progressing.

>> **Mind-Body Tip:** To get better leverage breathing in this exercise, instead of holding the opposite wrist, place the hand on your lower ribs on the side you're bending toward, and concentrate exhalations on moving your ribs inward under your hand.

Standing Side Bend

This exercise works to strengthen and stretch the obliques and quadratus lumborum (side waist and low side-back muscles) to promote proper rib movement and rib cage position to support optimal spine position and movement. It also trains healthy lateral mobility of the spine.

1. Stand with your feet hip-distance apart.

2. Inhale to raise your arms overhead. When you do, you will notice that your rib cage pushes forward and your low back arches.

3. Exhale and draw your lower ribs in, back, and down while also neutralizing your low back. Be sure you aren't arching your low back! You'll need to maintain a core contraction to hold this position with your arms overhead.

4. Inhale as you grab your right wrist with your left hand.

5. Exhale as you side bend to the left. Think about drawing your left lower ribs in as you exhale to contract your oblique muscles and help you actively side bend deeper. You should feel a stretch all the way through the right front of your hip, low back, and side of your body into your shoulder.

6. Take a total of 3 breaths while stretching to the left.

7. Return to center with your arms overhead. Repeat on the other side.

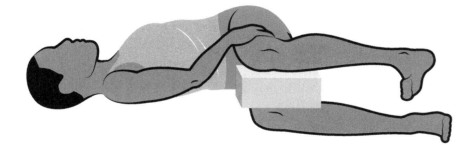

>> **Mind-Body Tip:** Imagine that your breathing is the engine of your twist; every inhale fills the space of your back to move your shoulders toward the floor while each exhale rotates your rib cage a little more.

Supine Double Bent-Knee Twist

Remember, not all twists work for people with back pain, but if done correctly they can help significantly. This exercise helps you focus on using your breathing and rib movement to support thoracic spine rotation and release of tension in the low back.

1. Lie on your right side with your knees bent at a 90-degree angle and stacked in front of your hips. Place a yoga block or pillow between your knees.

2. Place a pad or pillow under your head to keep your neck neutral.

3. Reach both hands out in line with your shoulders, laying your palms (left over right) together on the floor.

4. Inhale and look left as you open your left arm and shoulder to the left while keeping both knees in place on the right. Place your right hand on the outside of your left leg to help hold it in place, keeping your hips and knees stacked.

5. Twist from the middle of your back—not your low back. Exhale and focus on drawing your right lower ribs inward to help rotate your rib cage and thoracic spine further into the twist.

6. Take 2 more breaths, holding the position and continuing to focus on rib movement with the phases of your breath. Then release back to the start.

7. Gently flip over to repeat all the steps from the left side.

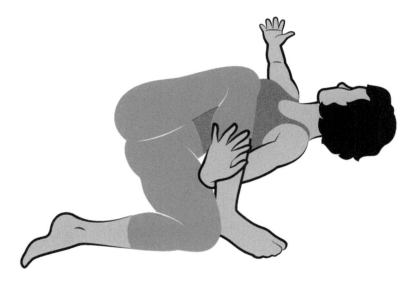

>> **Cautions:** If you experience any low-back pain in the twisting progression of this exercise, stick to the original Supine Figure-Four Stretch (page 57).

>> **Mind-Body Tip:** Focus your attention on the gentle pull of gravity enabling you to drop your hip open and release into the twist.

Supine Figure-Four Twist

This exercise adds a twist to the previous figure-four hip opener that creates thoracic rotation as well as an additional emphasis on the upper aspect of the outer hip area known as the TFL. Tension in this area not only leads to low-back pain but also painfully tight IT bands—the fascia on the outside of the leg.

1. Lie on your back with your knees bent and feet on the floor, hip-distance apart.

2. Bring your right leg up and place your right ankle on your left thigh above your left knee, creating a figure-four position.

3. Lift your left foot to bring your bent left knee toward your left shoulder, keeping it aligned.

4. Reach your hands around either side of your left thigh and clasp your hands together to hold your leg.

5. While still holding your legs in place, exhale as you roll to the left and place the right sole of the foot on the floor. There is no graceful way to do this—you will likely flop to the side.

6. Release your arms and place your left hand on the top of your right foot.

7. Inhale and reach your right arm out to the right at shoulder height.

8. Try to drop the right hip/glute down toward the mat to increase the outer-hip stretch.

9. Hold for 5 long, deep breaths. Unwind and repeat on other side.

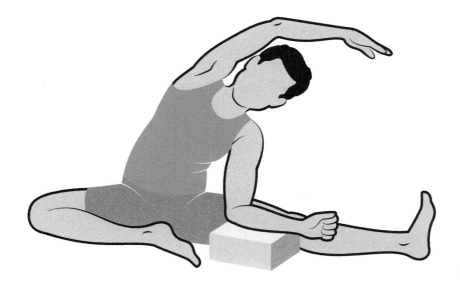

>> **Mind-Body Tip:** Tune into the differences in sensation you feel in your back as you move your top arm position so that you can control the amount of stretch and effort, as you deem appropriate.

Bent-Knee Straddle Stretch

The quadratus lumborum (mentioned in part 1 as one of the paired set of muscles supporting the spine) can get very tight, especially more so on one side than the other. It's therefore important to release that tension in order to find a more neutral position for your spine. In my experience, this is one of the safest and most effective ways to release it while also building core strength and stretching the hips and legs.

1. From a seated straddle position with both legs stretched out to the sides as wide as you comfortably can, bend your right knee and slide the sole of your right foot toward the inside of your left leg, up near your groin.

2. Place a foam block on the inside of your left leg and exhale as you side bend to the left to place your left forearm on top of it, parallel to your leg.

3. Inhale as you lift and reach your right arm up and over your head to the left, as shown.

4. Try moving the position of your arm (deeper or shallower into the stretch) and rotating your torso to find a "sweet spot" where you feel you are addressing the most tension in your right lower back/side waist.

5. Hold for another 2 to 3 breaths.

6. Release and repeat on the other side.

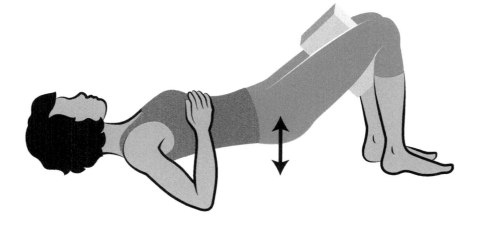

›› **Cautions:** This is a more difficult exercise than the regular Breathing Bridge (pages 69 and 111). If you feel pain or any cautionary sensation in your back during this exercise, replace it with any of the previous breathing exercises that have worked for you without causing pain.

›› **Mind–Body Tip:** Once you feel confident that you've mastered the muscle activation, concentrate on the synchronization with your breath to create a flowing pattern of movement.

Flowing Bridge

This is just like the Breathing Bridge (pages 69 and 111) exercise except it adds up-and-down movement synced with your breath. Adding the movement increases your ability to train for strengthening and body awareness as you focus on feeling your glutes and core fire to lift your hips in each repetition.

1. Begin on your back with your knees bent and feet on the floor hip-distance apart and about six inches from your bottom.

2. If necessary, use a folded towel or thin pillow under your head to keep your neck neutral. Don't use anything too big that bends your head forward or tucks your chin.

3. Place a foam yoga block, rolled towel, or pillow between your legs to engage the inner thighs (adductors) and avoid your hips externally rotating and knees splaying out.

4. With your arms at your sides, slide your shoulder blades down to relax your upper back and neck.

5. Place your hands on your lower ribs, so you can pay attention to and guide the movement of your ribs with your breathing.

6. On exhalation, as you draw your low ribs in and down toward your waist, engage your low, deep core to initiate lifting your hips a few inches off the floor. Avoid arching your low back.

7. Inhale for a count of 5 as you gently lower your hips to the floor. Exhale for a count of 7 as you lift your hips again. Repeat for a total of 5 breaths/repetitions.

8. Rest for a few breaths and repeat for another set of 5 breaths.

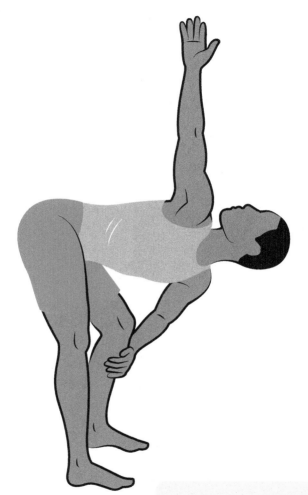

>> **Mind-Body Tip:** Initially, focus less on the twist and more on the sensations you feel in the back of your straight leg and side of your low back, ensuring that your lower body is stable enough to support deepening your twist.

Windmill Twist

Tight hamstrings are often blamed for hampering movement and causing pain, including back pain. However, the blame is usually misplaced since hamstring tension is generally caused by a misaligned pelvis pulling the hamstrings into a state of overuse. That said, addressing hamstring tension and pelvis position at the same time can provide back pain relief and prevention of recurrent tension. The Windmill Twist is a multipurpose posture that addresses the hamstrings and pelvis/hips while also stretching the quadratus lumborum on either side of the low back and training thoracic spine (mid-back) rotation to avoid low-back compensatory pain.

1. From standing with your feet hip-distance apart, exhale as you squat down and place your left hand on your left shin (as pictured).

2. Inhale as you reach your right arm forward and up, rotating from your shoulder, mid back, and rib cage to twist open to the right.

3. At the same time, straighten your right leg only (leaving your left knee bent) while pulling back through your heel like you're sliding it backward. You should experience a stretch in the back of your leg and across your right low back.

4. Hold for 5 breaths, using respiration to facilitate the twist. Focus inhalations on the open side of your rib cage (the side you're turning toward) and exhalations on the opposite side, employing side-waist muscles to internally rotate your ribs for greater rotation.

5. Unwind back to standing and repeat the movement with rotation to the left.

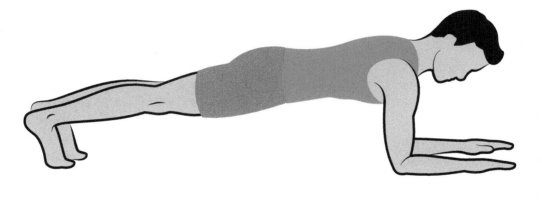

>> **Cautions:** If your core is initially too weak to hold the plank without your low back arching, decrease the length of your hold to 2 breaths and/or keep your knees down.

>> **Mind-Body Tip:** Zero in on the muscle activation needed to create this posture, segment by segment with strength and without pain.

Segmented Forearm Plank

Because this exercise requires core activation with a neutral spine, it helps strengthen and restore posture to combat back pain. Unlike a basic forearm plank, this segmented version eliminates typical compensation patterns, like pushing forward into the shoulders.

1. From a prone (on your belly) position with your forearms down and elbows directly under your shoulders, inhale as you lift only your rib cage. Exhale and pause in that position.

2. Inhale and lift your belly button, exhaling to hold that position.

3. Continue building the forearm plank position segment by segment with an inhale-to-lift, exhale-to-hold breathing pattern. Lift the front of your hips, pause, then lift your thighs all the way to your kneecaps. Finally, come up into a full forearm plank position by curling your toes under, lifting your knees, and straightening your legs.

4. Do not reposition or push weight forward into your arms. You should feel it most in your core.

5. Keep your low deep core engaged and rib cage pushed back to avoid collapsing through your belly and arching your back.

6. Hold the posture for 5 breaths or more.

7. To come out of the posture, reverse the sequence and the breathing pattern. Exhale as you bring only your knees back down. Inhale as you pause in that position. Exhale as you bring your thighs down, inhaling as you pause there. Continue to come down segment by segment until you return to your belly.

8. Repeat all the steps one more time for a total of 2 repetitions.

9. As you get stronger, increase how long you hold the position. Can you eventually hold for 10 breaths—or even 20—without letting your back sway?

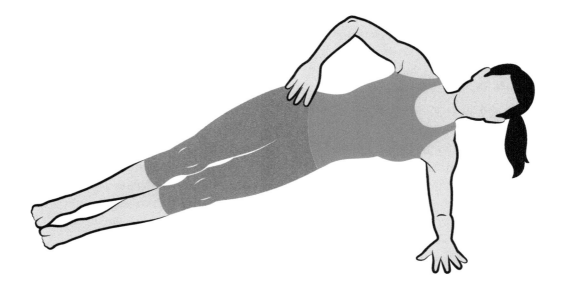

>> **Mind-Body Tip:** Don't lose track of shoulder alignment as you concentrate on oblique strength. Remain mindful of your shoulder's optimal position above your elbow.

Side Forearm Plank

The strength and function of your side-waist muscles, known as the obliques, are essential to rib cage positioning and rib movement during breathing as well as the ability of the thoracic spine to rotate. Consequently, they have an influence on overall back health and posture. This exercise focuses primarily on strengthening those muscles while also training stability through the shoulder girdle and pelvis.

1. Lie on a yoga mat or padded surface on your left side with your elbow directly under your shoulder and your legs extended. Place your left hand palm-down on the floor.

2. Stack your right foot on top of the left.

3. As you exhale, gently contract your abs and lift your hips and knees off the mat, keeping the side of your left foot and your left forearm and elbow in contact with the ground.

4. Take 5 long, deep breaths, focusing on exhales like oblique crunches to draw the lower ribs in back and down, contracting the side-waist and core muscles.

5. Repeat on your right side.

6. If you have a noticeable imbalance of strength (usually the left side is weaker), do another set on your weaker side.

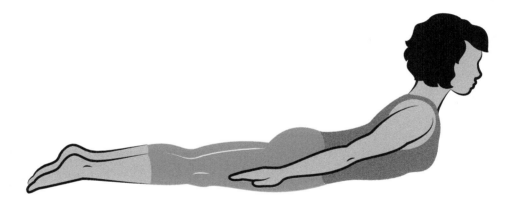

>> **Mind-Body Tip:** Never confuse muscular effort and cautionary strain. Be cautious and mindful in this strengthening exercise, and stop immediately if you experience any pain.

Locust

Like Sphinx with Head Turns (page 71) and Cobra (page 75), this posture activates the muscles of the back to hold the thoracic spine in extension. Taking away the support of the arms increases the difficulty and intensifies the strengthening aspect. Do not progress to this posture until you've comfortably mastered Cobra.

1. Lie prone (on your belly) on a yoga mat or padded surface with your arms along your sides and your legs and feet together. Keep the toes pointed back with the tops of your feet down on the mat (plantar flexion).

2. Without arching your low back (which would overuse the low-back extensors), lift your head, upper torso, and arms. You'll be resting on your lower ribs, belly, and front of your pelvis with your legs and the tops of your feet pressed to the floor.

3. Keep your arms straight and lifted, palms facing down, as you actively slide your shoulder blades down your back.

4. Your legs should remain close together. Hold a yoga block or pillow between your legs if they drift apart.

5. Gaze forward, being careful not to jut your chin forward and compress the back of your neck.

6. Hold for 3 to 5 breaths.

7. Exhale and rest for a breath or two with your right cheek and shoulders on the mat and your arms at your sides. Inhale and repeat the exercise. Then rest on the left cheek with your arms at your sides.

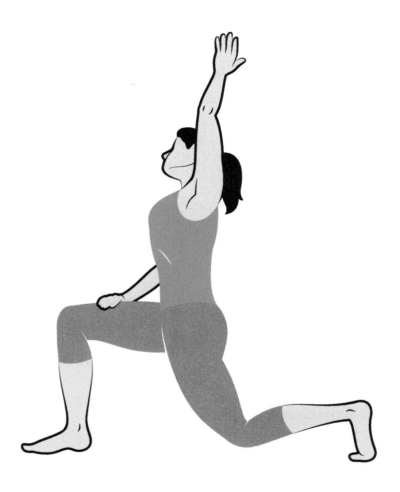

>> **Cautions:** If you experience discomfort when kneeling, place a folded towel or pad under your knee.

>> **Mind-Body Tip:** Knowing the connection between your psoas and diaphragm, use your exhales to deepen your reach and help stretch out your hip flexors.

Kneeling Lunge with Reach

This exercise combines the glute activation and hip flexor stretch you practiced in Kneeling Lunge (page 51) with the added side-body stretch you experienced in Gate Pose (page 53) and Supported Warrior Hip Flexor Stretch (page 45). It's a great way to open up areas that become compressed from too much sitting and contribute to poor posture and tight back muscles.

1. Set up in a kneeling lunge position on a yoga mat or slightly padded surface with your right leg in front and left leg behind. Add extra padding under your knee, if necessary for comfort.

2. Align both feet horizontally with your hips, and align your left knee directly below your left hip and your right knee directly above your right ankle.

3. Place your right hand on your right thigh for balance and support.

4. Inhale as you reach your left arm up and over in the same manner as in the Supported Warrior Hip Flexor Stretch (page 45), stretching your back laterally.

5. Exhale to drop the lower ribs in, back, and down, especially on the right side, which will increase your side bend. You should feel your left glute muscles engage to create an opposing stretching sensation in the front of your left hip.

6. Take 3 long, deep breaths in this position, focusing on the stretching sensation you feel in the front of your left hip and side body as your left glute remains engaged.

7. Switch sides and repeat.

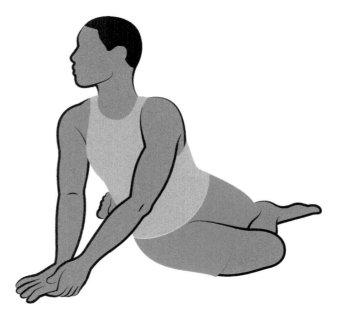

>> **Mind-Body Tip:** Don't let the complexity of the steps of this movement overwhelm you. Follow each instruction at your own pace to find your way comfortably into the exercise.

90/90 Seated Twist

As you progress through your program, decreasing pain and increasing strength and movement, you become ready for more complex movements that take you through multiple planes of motion and efficiently impact numerous areas at once. This is a variation of an exercise called the Bretzel 2.0 that I learned from Gray Cook, the renowned physical therapist and creator of Functional Movement Systems. When done properly, it opens the hips, enhances thoracic spine rotation, increases core strength and mobility, and releases overworked low-back muscles.

1. On a yoga mat or padded surface, sit on the outside of your right hip and leg with both knees bent at a 90-degree angle.

2. Your right knee and shin should be aligned in front of you, and although your weight is shifted to the right, you should still be facing forward with your shoulders parallel with your right shin.

3. Bring your left knee forward enough for the kneecap to touch your right heel.

4. Place your right hand on the floor for support, about six inches from your right hip.

5. Place your left hand on your left lower ribs as you exhale and guide them in, back, and down as you begin to rotate your torso to the right, turning your head to look over your right shoulder.

6. Inhale as you slide your left hand with the palm up underneath your right hand (as shown in the illustration).

7. Straighten both arms.

8. Take 4 more breaths for a total of 5. Focus on rotating from your middle back, using your breathing to help you. Inhale to expand in the right side of your rib cage and exhale to engage your core muscles on the left to help rotate your ribs in and to the right.

9. Unwind and set up to repeat the steps on the left.

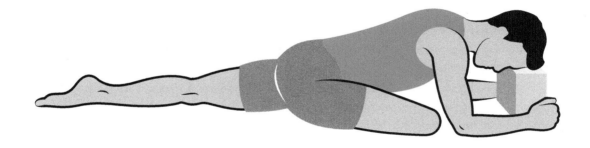

>> **Cautions:** You should not feel knee pain or any cautionary sensations in your knees. If you do, try bringing your front foot in closer to your body to decrease the angle of your shin. You can also place a prop, like a pillow or folded blanket, under the hip you're stretching. If those modifications don't work, this exercise is not appropriate for you.

>> **Mind-Body Tip:** You have control of the depth of this hip-opening exercise. Listen to your body so you can modify and progress according to your needs.

Pigeon

Pigeon is another widely known traditional yoga posture. It's a deep hip opener. Only progress to this position after you're fully comfortable with the Supine Figure-Four Twist (page 85) and you don't feel any added tension in your back or pulling sensation in your knees.

1. Starting on your hands and knees, bring your right knee forward and place it behind your right wrist. Slide your right foot up behind your left wrist. The more your right leg is parallel with the front of your mat, the more intense the hip opener will be.

2. Slide your left leg behind you, straightening your knee and pointing your toes back.

3. Gently lower your hips, taking care to keep your pelvis level.

4. On an exhale, walk your hands forward on the fingertips and lower your upper body to the floor. If you can come low enough, rest your forehead on the floor with your arms outstretched. Otherwise, rest your forehead on your stacked fists or on a yoga block.

5. Stay here for 5 long, deep breaths, using exhalations to focus your attention on releasing tension in your right hip.

6. Come out of the pose by pushing back through your hands to lift your hips and move your legs back into an all-fours position.

7. Repeat on the other side.

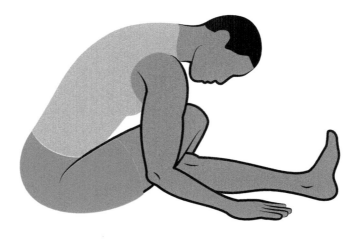

>> **Cautions:** If you feel any cautionary discomfort in your low back while in this posture, don't do it!

>> **Mind-Body Tip:** Move slowly and carefully into this stretch, being mindful of where and how you feel the sensation in your legs, backing off if it becomes too much or moves into your back.

Seated Hamstring and Hip Stretch

Tight hamstrings and hips can lead to compensation through the low back. This exercise addresses such tightness. However, it can be a very significant hamstring stretch, so go into it gently and with awareness. Don't force the stretch.

1. On a yoga mat or padded surface, sit with both legs straight out in front of you.

2. Bend your right knee and cross your right foot over your straight left leg.

3. Point your right toes and try to slide your foot back toward your left hip.

4. If needed, hold your leg in place with your hands. If your top leg is pushing uncomfortably on your bottom leg, you can place a folded towel in between them. Inhale and sit tall.

5. Exhale and hinge from the hips to fold your upper body over your legs as deeply as you can without pain.

6. You should feel a significant stretch through the back of your left leg as well as some stretching sensation through your right hip.

7. If you aren't using your hands to hold your bent leg in place, walk your hands forward on either side of your straight leg.

8. Keep the foot of your left leg dorsiflexed (toes pointing up).

9. Hold for 3 breaths.

10. Repeat the exercise with the left leg on top.

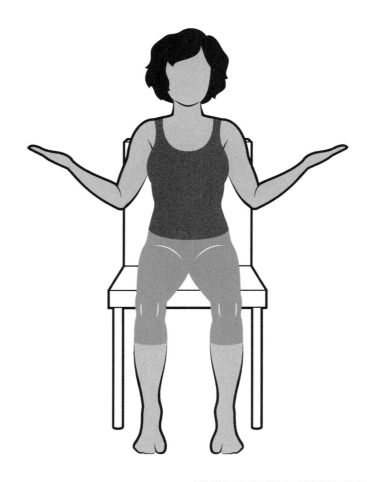

>> **Mind-Body Tip:** Although it takes a little effort to put yourself into a "good" posture, once it's established, let yourself relax and find ease without losing the position.

Seated Posture Exercise with 10-Breath Breathing Break

The simplest and most effective way to correct your posture is to use something called "reciprocal inhibition," which is a term that describes how muscles work together in opposing pairs. By activating underused muscles in your mid back to pull your shoulder blades down, you can turn off the overactive muscles in your upper back, chest, and neck that pull you forward into a slouch.

1. Sit in a chair with both feet firmly on the ground and your weight centered evenly between your two sitting bones, the pair of bony ischial tuberosities of the pelvis you can feel on either side when you sit.

2. Hold your arms out in front of you at shoulder height with your palms up.

3. Inhale and open your arms out to your sides, keeping your shoulders down and your neck long.

4. Exhale as you bend your elbows and lower them toward the sides of your body, keeping your palms up. Use the muscles on the outside of your upper rib cage and base of your shoulder blades (serratus and lower traps) to slide your shoulder blades downward. This will automatically shut off your overactive neck and chest muscles to open your shoulders and chest.

5. Drop your chin down and back until it feels level, while aligning your head and neck between your shoulders.

6. Once you feel you are optimally positioned, without losing the posture you've established, gently lay your hands in your lap.

7. From your state of optimal posture, focus your mind entirely on breathing and count 10 long, deep breaths.

CHAPTER 5

Exercises for Maintenance and Prevention

Now that you're out of pain and you have built up the strength and mobility to sustain a healthy back, it's important to practice maintenance to prevent future issues.

Remember the statistic that 80 percent of people who suffer one episode of acute back pain end up with another? The content of this chapter is meant to counter that stat.

I've outlined 10 exercises for you. The first three should be practiced daily, leaving you with seven additional exercises to be done at least three times per week. The remaining seven exercises in this chapter are only suggestions. It's up to you to select your own "lucky seven" to integrate into your overall exercise regimen to ensure you're maintaining functional movement through all planes of motion while continuing to cultivate strength, recovery, and a healthy mind-body connection. Within the introduction to each of the seven suggested exercises, I reference similar exercises covered in the previous chapters, so you can decide what works best for you.

Because you've been building a strong mind-body connection throughout this process, trust your instincts to choose the exercises that you find most effective. Also, listen to your body so you'll know if or when it's time to go back and practice exercises from earlier chapters to rebuild strength and mobility or help alleviate any discomfort that may arise from time to time. You should feel empowered to be proactive and confident in your own self-care!

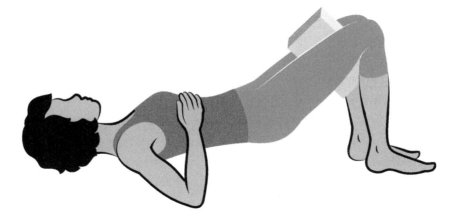

>> **Mind-Body Tip:** Breathing is your life force. Keep in mind that with every opportunity you have to train your breathing, you're strengthening much more than just respiration.

Breathing Bridge

At this point, you should have mastered this exercise and be practicing it every day. This is the starting position that all of my athletes use to train their breathing during warm-ups.

1. Begin on your back on a yoga mat or padded surface, with your knees bent and feet on the floor hip-distance apart and about six inches from your bottom.

2. If necessary, use a folded towel or thin pillow under your head to keep your neck neutral. Don't use anything too big that bends your head forward or tucks your chin.

3. Place a foam yoga block, rolled towel, or pillow between your legs to engage the inner thighs (adductors) and avoid your hips externally rotating and knees splaying out.

4. With your arms at your sides, slide your shoulder blades down to relax your upper back and neck.

5. Place your hands on your lower ribs so you can pay attention to and guide the movement of your ribs with your breathing.

6. On an exhalation, as you draw your low ribs in and down toward your waist, engage your low, deep core to initiate lifting your hips a few inches off the floor, as you did in Breathing Bridge on Chair (page 49). Avoid arching your low back.

7. While bridging, inhale through your nose, filling the lowest lobes of your lungs. You should feel your lower ribs externally rotate to expand outward, as opposed to only inflating your upper chest.

8. Exhale, using core muscles to help internally rotate your lower ribs and release your rib cage downward, expelling all air. A complete exhalation is necessary to fully relax your diaphragm.

9. Take 5 long, deep breaths at a 5-count inhale, 7-count exhale while holding your bridge position. At the end of each exhale, pause without taking a breath for a count of 3. Ideally, your breathing count should be 7 inhale, 9 exhale, and 3- to 5-count pause.

10. After 5 breaths, release from the bridge, rest a moment, and repeat for another set of 5 breaths.

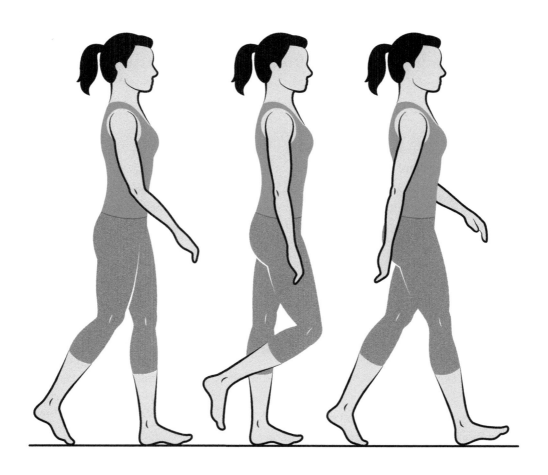

>> **Mind-Body Tip:** Once you feel comfortable with the mechanics of your gait, walking can begin to feel like meditation in motion. Notice and appreciate how your body was designed to move.

Walking with Awareness of Gait Mechanics

If you were listening to an orchestra and the trombone was playing an unplanned solo while the other instruments tried to figure out how to cover it up, it wouldn't sound very good. The muscles of your body work together like an orchestra; one errant trombone can ruin the music. If walking has been painful for you in the past, it's likely that muscles that have been compensating and contributing to your back pain are to blame. By mindfully training your gait (walking) pattern to be a symphony in motion, you'll be able to initiate and maintain healthy movement to prevent future pain.

Walking is an alternating and reciprocal pattern, which simply means that while one side of the body is doing one thing, the other is doing the exact opposite to create a complete movement. This includes both the upper and lower halves of our bodies and incorporates all the supporting spinal muscles addressed in previous chapters. Correct foot position and heel strike will enable you to absorb shock and move the load of your weight with balance and control. Arm swing is often overlooked but it's essential to a functional walking pattern because it creates healthy movement of the rib cage in coordination with each step, facilitating the necessary core, hip, and trunk power that prevents stress on the spine.

Because our bodies are designed for walking and it's a necessary part of living for able-bodied individuals, it's recommended that we take 10,000 steps per day. As part of your maintenance program, I recommend at least 10 minutes of mindful walking each day. As you take each step, be aware of the synchronicity of all the movements involved and your ability to breathe well as you walk.

Continued

1. As you take your first step with your right foot, your heel should make contact first, then the sole, moving into your toes as your heel lifts, bringing you forward to your toes to begin to take another step.

2. At the same time that your forward right heel strikes, your back left foot should be pushing off the toes.

3. Feet should point forward as you walk, with no duck feet, which can signal open hips and an improperly positioned pelvis that will put more stress on your back.

4. When you're walking, arm and leg position should oppose each other on the same side. For example, when the right foot is moving forward, the right arm is swinging back and the left arm is swinging forward with the left leg in back.

5. Walk for at least 10 minutes every day. You don't need to think about your gait pattern the entire time you are walking, but check in on it from time to time to ensure that it is smooth and following the pattern outlined above.

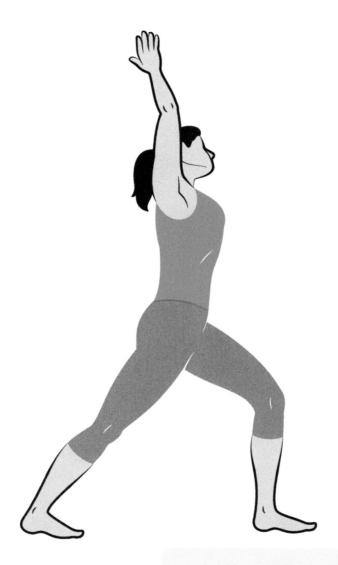

>> **Mind-Body Tip:** This is a powerful exercise to counter the impact of prolonged sitting. Be mindful of how you hold your body throughout the day so you'll remember to practice this stretch proactively.

Warrior Hip Flexor Stretch

Unlike the supported variation of this you did in the initial set of exercises in chapter 3, this version adds an element of balance, which requires use of the core strength you built with the exercises in chapter 4. It still stretches out hip flexors and side-waist and low-back muscles to alleviate any built-up tension from sitting that could lead to back pain. This is my go-to move whenever I get up from my desk, get out of the car after a long drive, or whenever I can stand on an airplane. You should be doing this at least once a day, if not more, depending on how much time you spend sitting and traveling.

1. From a standing position, step your right foot back, as though coming into a lunge, but place your heel down with your toes angled slightly out. Bend your left knee to align it above your left ankle, keeping your back leg straight.

2. Place your left hand on your left hip. If balance is a challenge, place your left hand on a wall or other support, as you did with this exercise in chapter 3; otherwise, try to do it unsupported, using core strength for balance.

3. Inhale as you lift your right arm up and over your head.

4. Exhale as you side bend to the left. Avoid arching your lower back.

5. As you hold the position, press the front of your right hip forward (like you are trying to tuck your tailbone under you) to release your right hip flexors.

6. Hold for 3 long, deep breaths. Repeat on the other side.

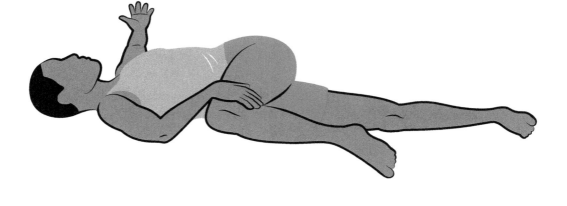

>> **Cautions:** If twisting felt cautionary in the previous chapter, continue to approach all rotational exercises with extreme care. Never force rotation. If you experience any pain or cautionary sensations, back off.

>> **Mind-Body Tip:** If this twist works for you, incorporate a visualization to increase its tension-releasing effect. Imagine your body like a damp washcloth, and the twist gently wringing out all the water.

Supine Single-Leg, Bent-Knee Twist

If twisting exercises worked for you while regaining your strength and mobility, then they should be part of your maintenance program. Feel free to incorporate any of the twists you liked from the previous chapter: Windmill Twist (page 91), Supine Double Bent-Knee Twist (page 83), Supine Figure-Four Twist (page 85), Seated Bent-Knee Twist (page 77), or 90/90 Seated Twist (page 101). This new twist is a gentle alternative to the Supine Double Bent-Knee Twist. However, without proper body awareness, it's easy to twist from your low back rather than your mid back. When done correctly, this exercise stretches hip, groin, and low-back muscles while enhancing mid-back mobility and increasing blood flow in the pelvis and abdomen.

1. Lie on your back on a yoga mat or padded surface with your legs extended and arms at your sides. Place a thin pillow under your head, if desired.

2. Hug both knees evenly into your chest, and interlace your fingers around your left knee.

3. Inhale as you straighten your right leg, pushing your heel skyward.

4. Exhale as you slowly lower your right leg down to the floor in line with your hip. Use your core muscles to control your leg's descent and avoid arching your low back as you lower the leg.

5. Inhale as you place your right hand on the outside of your left thigh and reach your left arm to the left.

6. Exhale fully as you gently twist from your mid back (*not* your low back) to bring your left knee across your body to the right.

7. Take 2 more long, deep breaths, focusing exhales on the right side of your rib cage where the ribs are closing in and inhales on the more open left side of the rib cage, facilitating your twist.

8. Unwind and repeat on the other side.

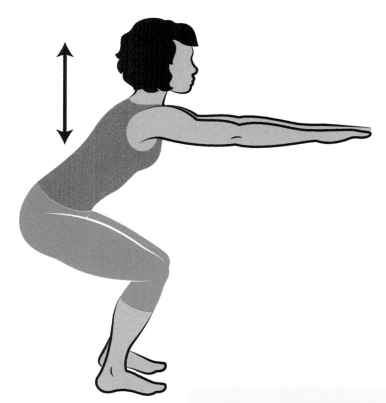

>> **Mind-Body Tip:** This is actually a movement you practice in some form multiple times per day (anytime you sit down and stand up). But by doing it mindfully, synchronized with your breath, you turn it into a controlled strengthening and flowing exercise.

Flowing Chair Squat

When done correctly, this is a strengthening exercise for all the supporting muscles of your spine, including not only back muscles but also core, glute, and leg muscles. Other exercises covered previously that address similar areas include Roll-Into-a-Ball Core Exercise (page 73), Segmented Forearm Plank (page 93), and Bent-Knee Down Dog with Pedal Out (page 79).

1. From a standing position with feet hip-distance apart, establish a breathing pattern of a 5-count inhale and a 5-count exhale.

2. Exhale as you drop your rib cage, engage your core, and sit back into a gentle squatting position with your arms straight out in front at shoulder height.

3. Inhale as you raise your arms overhead, and keep them shoulder-distance apart while you come back up to standing.

4. Do not allow your feet to turn out; keep them planted with toes pointed forward. Press through your heels to use your glute, core, and leg muscles to power up from the squat to standing.

5. If you have trouble feeling your glutes and core working in this posture, try it with a chair behind you and lightly touch your bottom down on the chair seat (without releasing your full weight onto the chair) before pushing back up to standing.

6. Repeat the movement for a total of five times, flowing with a breathing pattern of a 5-count inhale and a 5-count exhale, exhaling into the squat and inhaling to stand with arms overhead.

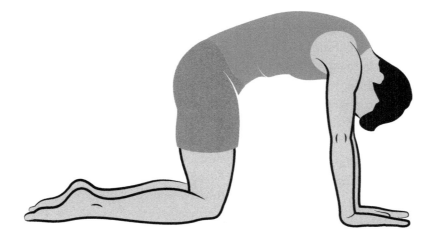

>> **Cautions:** If you've had spinal fusion surgery, parts of your spine may be unable to move well, so don't force it. If you experience any pain, do not practice this exercise.

Cat Flow

Because this exercise trains your mind-body connection while also training a controlled full range of spinal flexion and extension, it's one of my favorite maintenance exercises. However, as an alternative, you can use two of the previous exercises, Cobra (page 75) and Roll-Into-a-Ball Core Exercise (page 73), to work both of the back-bending movements done in Cat Flow.

1. Begin on your hands and knees with your hips stacked directly above your knees, ankles aligned horizontally with your feet, shoulders directly above your wrists, and head neutral, looking at the floor.

2. Inhale and imagine your spine as a long strand of pearls that you can articulate, pearl by pearl, starting from your tailbone.

3. Exhale as you tilt your pelvis under to tuck your tailbone to begin taking the shape of a big, angry cat, flexing your entire spine. Create the flexion, segment by segment, stretching your lower back and then continuing to your mid back and, finally, your neck and head. You should feel like your core is engaged and your rib cage is pushed as far back in your body as possible to support the flexion of your spine.

4. As you inhale, start again at your tailbone, tilting it up to gently arch your low back and letting that arch move into your mid back and then to your neck and finally lifting the head to look straight forward. Notice that your head wants to move first, but don't let it. Practice body awareness and control by moving from tailbone to head with full control.

5. Repeat for a total of 5 breaths—exhaling into the rounded-back "angry" cat posture and inhaling into the arched-back "frisky" cat posture.

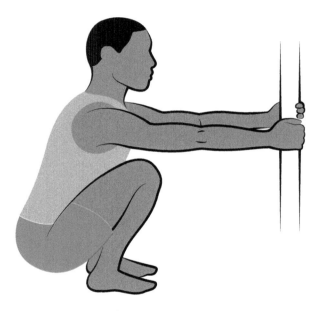

>> **Cautions:** If you have knee issues, be careful because deep knee bending is required for this posture. It's not unusual to feel light-headed upon standing after a round of these. Just continue to hold on to the secure structure and breathe normally until the feeling passes.

>> **Mind-Body Tip:** Focus on pushing your rib cage back to help round and lengthen your spine as you use your inhalations to expand your rib cage out and back, spreading and releasing your back muscles.

Supported Back-Release Squat

Unlike the Flowing Chair Squat (page 121), this exercise is intended to create more of a stretch throughout the back. Alternatives for releasing tight back muscles in a similar fashion are Child's Pose (page 41) or Child's Pose with Reach (page 59).

1. Stand with your feet hip-distance apart and your arms extended forward at shoulder level. Hold on to a pole, door frame, or other secure structure that reaches high enough and low enough to perform the exercise, as shown in the illustration.

2. Exhale and drop back through your hips and pelvis into a deep squat, walking your hands down the pole as you lower.

3. Maintain weight in your heels with your toes pointed forward. Don't let your feet or knees turn out or heels lift. If you experience discomfort in your ankles, knees, or shins, make sure you're dropping back into your hips as opposed to pushing forward into your knees. You should literally feel like your body weight is hanging off the pole, pushing back into your hips and heels.

4. Take 5 long, deep breaths. Focus inhalations on breathing into your mid back and exhalations on letting your lower back release. Stand and rest a moment, then repeat for another set of 5 breaths.

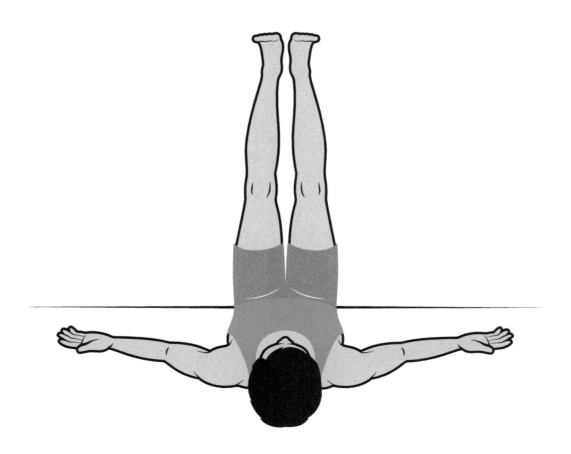

>> **Mind-Body Tip:** Focus your attention on the lightness of your feet and legs as they rest up the wall. Let the sensation be symbolic of letting go (at least temporarily) of any heavy burdens you might be carrying.

Legs Up the Wall

Some variation of this posture should definitely be part of your "lucky seven" exercises for maintenance and prevention. It's important to make time for resting and recovery. A few times a week, either throw your legs up the wall for the full posture (which gives you the bonus of a hamstring stretch) or simply get them up above your heart on a chair or large pillow. You'll reduce tension and swelling in your lower body while releasing your lower back. And you'll give your mind some quiet time. No scrolling through social media while in this posture—put down your phone!

1. Sit on the floor with your right shoulder and right hip a few inches from the wall.

2. Lower your left shoulder toward the floor and gently swing your legs straight up the wall with your back and head resting on the ground.

3. If having your legs straight up is too much for you, modify by moving farther away from the wall or resting your legs on a chair seat with your knees bent.

4. If you experience discomfort in your neck or back, place a thin pillow or folded blanket behind your head and/or hips.

5. Remain in this posture for 10 long, deep breaths, or longer, if you find it particularly effective. Because this is a favorite of mine, I usually spend 2 to 5 minutes in it.

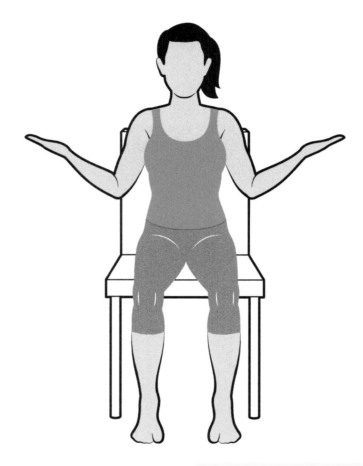

>> **Mind-Body Tip:** Research shows that holding your body in good posture with your chest and shoulders open not only feels good physically but also makes us feel more confident, happy, and at ease.

Seated Posture Exercise with 10-Breath Breathing Break

This is another exercise that I recommend as being one of your "lucky seven" maintenance exercises, if not one you do daily. Practicing this will not only reinforce good posture but also will positively influence your gait mechanics while walking. It will also make you more comfortable during times when you have to sit for prolonged periods.

1. Sit in a chair with both feet firmly on the ground and your weight centered evenly between your two sitting bones (the bony ischial tuberosities of the pelvis you can feel on either side when you sit).

2. Place your arms out in front of you at shoulder height with your palms up.

3. Inhale and open your arms out to your sides, keeping your shoulders down and your neck long.

4. Exhale as you bend your elbows down and in toward the sides of your body, your palms still up. Use the muscles on the outside of your upper rib cage and base of your shoulder blades (serratus and lower traps) to slide your shoulder blades downward. This will automatically shut off your overactive neck and chest muscles to open your shoulders and chest.

5. Drop your chin down and back until it feels level while aligning your head and neck between your shoulders.

6. Once you feel you are optimally positioned, without losing the posture you've established, gently lay your hands in your lap.

7. From your state of optimal posture, focus your mind entirely on breathing and count 10 long, deep breaths.

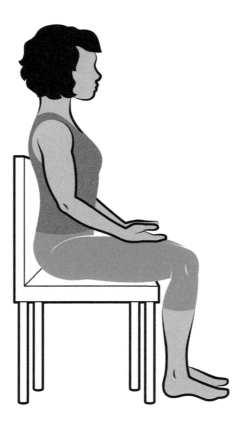

>> **Mind-Body Tip:** Even if practicing compassion weren't shown to help ease back pain (which it is), it's worth doing simply to be happier, as additional research shows that it makes us feel more satisfied with our lives.

Compassion Meditation

Throughout this program, you've learned that meditation isn't really that difficult or complex, and can pay big dividends in terms of pain and stress relief. A 2015 study at Stanford University found a significant correlation between pain relief and cultivating compassion through compassion-focused meditation, which is why I recommend incorporating this meditation focused on loving-kindness into your maintenance program.

1. Spend a moment to memorize this set of three phrases, repeating them silently: "May you be healthy in body and mind. May you be pain-free. May you be grateful and happy."

2. Review the following order of instructions so you'll be able to move through the sequence of the meditation without needing to overthink it.

3. Settle into a relaxed and comfortable position sitting, standing, or lying down.

4. Close your eyes and bring your attention to your breath, lengthening and deepening it to a comfortable pace.

5. Now bring your attention to your mind's eye (your imagination) and create the image of someone who loves you. This person could be living or passed. Visualize that person standing beside you, sending you warm wishes and love. Spend a moment feeling the warmth,

kindness, and compassion coming to you from that person.

6. Now turn your attention from receiving to giving. Focus on sending the love that you feel back to that person. Just like you, this person wishes to be happy.

7. Repeat your memorized phrases 3 times, silently: "May you be healthy in body and mind. May you be pain-free. May you be grateful and happy."

8. Now think of an acquaintance, someone you don't know very well. This could be a neighbor, the clerk you see regularly at your grocery store, or anyone else whose features you can clearly imagine but with whom you don't have a particularly intimate connection.

9. Remember that you and this person are alike in your desire for a good life.

Continued

10. Send them your wishes for well-being, repeating your set of phrases 3 times, silently: "May you be healthy in body and mind. May you be pain-free. May you be grateful and happy."

11. Now expand your awareness and picture the entire world as a globe in front of you. Imagine you could reach all people, everywhere, all of them, like you, wanting a good life.

12. Send them your warm wishes by repeating your phrases 3 times, silently: "May you be healthy in body and mind. May you be pain-free. May you be grateful and happy."

13. Bring your focus back to your breath, taking a few more long, deep breaths before gently reopening your eyes.

CHAPTER 6

Additional Therapies
for Back Pain

The American College of Physicians recommends acupuncture, massage, tai chai, and yoga, among other alternative therapies for back pain relief, and only turning to drugs or surgery when these types of treatments don't work. I agree with that approach; a well-rounded treatment and prevention plan should include these therapies whenever possible.

However, insurance doesn't always pay for alternative therapies, making them cost-prohibitive for many people with back pain. That's one of the reasons I've incorporated aspects of them into the self-care exercises in this book. That said, if your insurance covers these therapies or you are able to pay, it's in your best interest to leverage these therapies in conjunction with the exercises and knowledge you have learned in this book, to help relieve your pain and boost your back health. Below, I've outlined the pros and cons of some of the most common therapy options to help you determine what might work for you.

Physical Therapy (PT) uses a combination of techniques for reducing pain and restoring function. To be licensed, physical therapists are required to have an extensive education including at least a graduate degree, but many have doctoral degrees. PTs use a variety of techniques for relieving pain, including heat/cold and massage, but they primarily rely on corrective exercises directed at eliminating the cause of your pain. Many of the exercises in chapters 3 and 4 are modeled after a physical therapy approach since PT is best used to relieve pain and correct the cause.

Thankfully, PT is generally covered, at least in part, by most insurance plans for a certain number of visits each year. And most doctors specializing in back pain are associated with a physical therapist or two and can provide a referral. Some progressive doctors have physical therapists on staff as part of their practice. If your insurance company covers PT, it will be able to direct you to an in-network provider.

Yoga is a philosophy rooted in Hinduism and composed of a system of various practices designed to heighten spirituality. However, the popular Americanized versions of yoga offered in studios and gym settings are more secular forms of mind-body exercise and are focused more on breathing and movement exercises for mental and physical benefits, not spirituality. Many exercises in this book are yoga-inspired in nature but offered more from a corrective exercise approach.

Because styles of yoga can be wildly different, ranging from gentle to advanced power classes, and because yoga instructors aren't held to any education or certification standard, going to just any yoga class is unadvisable. As much as yoga is shown in studies to be an exercise style that can provide back pain relief, back pain from yoga injuries is also a common complaint in US emergency rooms. For that reason, use caution when selecting a yoga class, stick with classes labeled "gentle" or "restorative," and consider hiring a well-educated, experienced private yoga instructor specializing in back pain clients.

Pilates is similar to yoga with its focus on breathing and movement but has a greater concentration on core training and tends to be more physically demanding. And unlike yoga's five-thousand-year history as a spiritual practice, Pilates was developed in the twentieth century by Joseph Pilates as an exercise regimen done both on a mat and a large apparatus called a reformer.

Because of its emphasis on strengthening the core, Pilates can be beneficial in countering back pain in people with weak abdominal muscles. However, like yoga, it's not usually covered by insurance and your best application of it is with private lessons with a certified instructor who specializes in back pain relief and prevention. Several of the core exercises in this book are modeled after Pilates-based exercises.

Tai Chi is an ancient Chinese noncompetitive martial art that has evolved into a form of mind-body exercise often considered to be "meditation in motion." It involves a series of movements gracefully performed in a slow, focused manner coordinated with a deep breathing pattern. Several of the studies referenced in this book show that tai chi can be beneficial in helping back pain patients find relief. Unlike yoga and Pilates, this less intense form of exercise has a very low risk of injury.

Massage Therapy is the manual manipulation of soft body tissues (muscle and connective tissue) with the goal of releasing tension and improving circulation and muscle extensibility to alleviate pain and enhance movement. There are dozens of types of massage therapy modalities, and, depending on the cause of your back pain, many can serve as excellent treatments although some may not. The quality of your massage is also dictated by the education and experience of your therapist. Most states have licensing programs for massage therapists that require a minimum level of education and training, so you always want to ensure that your therapist is licensed.

Some insurance plans include partial coverage or a certain number of massage therapy visits with a back pain diagnosis, so don't assume it isn't covered without checking with your plan. If covered, your insurance will provide referrals. Otherwise, look for a licensed therapist experienced in massage techniques for back pain relief. Often, your doctor or PT will be able to refer you.

Self-Myofascial Release (SMR) is essentially comprised of self-massage techniques to accomplish the same benefits as regular massage therapy. Myofascial simply refers to the fascia (connective tissue) surrounding muscles. Foam rolling is probably the most common form of SMR. Foam rollers are large, firm cylinders that you lean on to roll parts of your body over to release tension and improve circulation.

I foam roll daily as part of my warm-up before exercise. I also travel with a compact foam roller to roll out tight muscles and promote circulation after long airplane or car rides. You can purchase foam rollers in most large department stores, sporting goods stores, or online for anywhere from $25 for compact foam construction to $150-plus for high-tech, vibrating rollers. Searching online, you'll find many articles with instructions for rolling out your body; you can find one I wrote for CNN called "Stave Off Soreness Like a Pro Athlete." As with any self-care exercises, use caution and listen to your body to determine what feels right for you.

Chiropractic Care is administered by a chiropractic doctor who uses spinal adjustment techniques to treat back pain without drugs or surgery. Chiropractors perform spinal adjustments by applying precise force directly to specific spine segments to enable movement and restore nerve function, which can alleviate pain and help maintain spine health. Most of the professional sports teams I work with have team chiropractors who adjust many of the players on a regular basis, working in concert with the team coaches, trainers, and PTs. The athletes I know who get adjusted regularly swear by it. That said, some people are uncomfortable with chiropractic care and feel it can be unsafe because the spinal adjustments can feel extreme and are often accompanied with loud cracking and popping sounds.

Because of the concerns associated with chiropractic care, and given that the quality of care and safety is dictated by the expertise of the practitioner, it is wise to research reviews or get a good referral from a trusted source familiar with the chiropractic doctor you are considering. Many large insurance plans offer some degree of coverage for chiropractic care (partial or a certain number of visits, for example), so check with your provider.

Acupuncture is a holistic treatment option that is a form of traditional Chinese medicine where thin needles are inserted into the skin to stimulate specific points on the body. A centuries-old practice, acupuncture is based on the theory that the body has energy pathways, known as meridians, that can become blocked by injury or illness and need to be reopened to restore balance and better health. Dry needling, also known as intramuscular stimulation (IMS), is a more modern, Westernized version of acupuncture. Rather than using meridians, needles are inserted into muscle trigger points to stimulate and restore normal function.

Studies have shown that both traditional acupuncture and dry needling can be useful adjunct pain-relief therapies. Unfortunately, most insurance plans don't cover acupuncture. If your plan does or you're able to pay, be sure to find a licensed practitioner with a good reputation. Sometimes, physical therapists or back pain doctors are also licensed in acupuncture. Thankfully, that was my experience when I hurt my back the last time, and my doctor was able to use acupuncture as one of the first treatments to help alleviate my pain and restore movement, so I could begin self-care exercises.

Mindfulness Meditation is a Westernized evolution of the 2,500-year-old practice of Buddhist "insight" meditation. It's a form of meditation designed to help us attune to the present moment and be able to observe and accept our inner and outer experiences with greater patience and compassion. Studies abound that point to mindfulness meditation as a highly effective means of relieving chronic back pain. One such study looked at brain scans of regular meditators and found increased activity in areas of the brain that regulate emotion and decreased activity in regions associated with pain.

Although you can find meditation coaches and yoga instructors who specialize in meditation, it is not difficult to practice on your own. All the exercise chapters in this book include mindfulness meditation exercises, and I urge you to continue this practice

as part of your health maintenance program, not only for your back, but also for the overall quality of your life. There are many meditation apps available for free or a small fee that you can use on your phone or computer for daily guided practices.

Cognitive Behavioral Therapy (CBT) is a psychotherapy that focuses on the development of coping strategies to change behaviors and emotional reactions to negative stimuli like pain, memories, negative thoughts, and so on. This therapy works to establish new patterns of thinking that train the brain away from pain and negative thinking to promote a better mood, positive actions, and reduced suffering. It was originally developed for treating depression but has been found effective for a number of conditions, including PTSD and pain management.

Like mindfulness meditation, studies have shown that CBT is effective in altering the gray matter of the brain that impacts pain modulation. Licensed mental health counselors, psychologists, psychotherapists, and psychiatrists can provide this type of therapy.

Most insurance programs offer mental health benefits that would at least partially, if not completely, cover CBT sessions.

Whether you pursue additional therapies for back pain or not, I hope that you've worked through all the exercise chapters to create an effective self-care program that has moved you out of pain and will help prevent pain in the future. It's been my goal to empower you with the education and means to proactively take care of your back. I hope we've accomplished that goal together, and I wish you continued health and happiness.

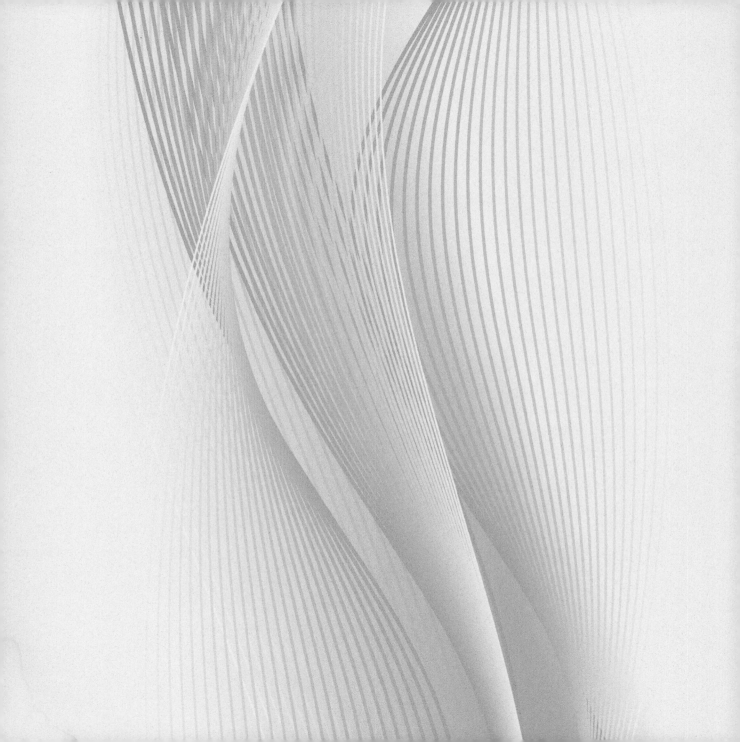

RESOURCES

American Chiropractic Association
    www.acatoday.org
American Massage Therapy Association
    www.amtamassage.org
American Physical Therapy Association
    www.apta.org
American Psychology Association
    www.apa.org
Functional Movement Systems
    www.functionalmovement.com
Happify.com
Hyperice Vibrating Foam Rollers
    & SMR tools and info: www.hyperice.com
Postural Restoration Institute
    www.posturalrestoration.com
YogaAlliance.org

These are some of my related CNN articles:
www.cnn.com/2015/04/07/health/athlete
    -soreness-yoga/index.html
www.cnn.com/2016/03/24/health/back-exercise
    -pain-prevention-yoga/index.html
www.cnn.com/2015/10/08/health/breathe-like
    -pro-athlete
www.cnn.com/2014/08/19/health/sciatica-pain
    -relief-yoga/index.html
www.cnn.com/2016/11/03/health/yoga-stress
    -strategies/index.html

REFERENCES

Ahmed, Abdul-Kareem. "Cognitive Behavioral Therapy Changes Gray Matter Morphology in Chronic Pain." (Nov. 25, 2013). *Pain Research Forum.* www.painresearchforum.org/news /34218-cognitive-behavioral-therapy-changes -gray-matter-morphology-chronic-pain.

American Chiropractic Association. "Back Pain Facts and Statistics." Accessed Nov. 17, 2017. www.acatoday.org/Patients/Health-Wellness -Information/Back-Pain-Facts-and-Statistics.

Bernstein, Robert M., Harold Cozen. "Evaluation of Back Pain in Children and Adolescents." *America Family Physician* 76 no. 11: (December 2007). www.aafp.org/afp/2007/1201 /p1669.html.

Brandt, Steve. "Wandering mind not a happy mind." Harvard gazette (blog). (November 11, 2010). www.news.harvard.edu/gazette /story/2010/11/wandering-mind-not-a -happy-mind.

Calais-Germain, Blandine. *Anatomy of Breathing.* Seattle, WA: Eastland Press Inc., 2006.

Centers for Disease Control and Prevention. "Vital signs: overdoses of prescription opioid pain relievers—United States, 1999–2008." 60 no. 43 (Nov. 11, 2017): 1487–92. *CDC Morbidity and Mortality Weekly Report.*

Cherkin, Daniel C., Karen J. Sherman, Benjamin H. Balderson, Andrea J. Cook, Melissa L. Anderson, Renee J. Hawkes, Kelly E. Hansen, Judith A. Turner. "Effect of Mindfulness-Based Stress Reduction vs. Cognitive Behavioral Therapy or Usual Care on Back Pain and Functional Limitations in Adults with Chronic Low Back Pain: A Randomized Clinical Trial." *JAMA* 315 no. 12 (March 2016): 1240–49. doi: 10.1001/jama/.2016.2323.

Darnall, Beth D. "Compassion Cultivation in Chronic Pain May Reduce Anger, Pain, and Increase Acceptance: Study Review and Brief

Commentary." *Health Care Current Review* 3 no. 2 (Oct. 20, 2015): 142. doi: 10.4172/2375 -4273.1000142.

Donahue, Louise. "7 Back Pain Conditions That Mainly Affect Women." (Updated Nov. 17, 2016). *Spine-health.* www.spine-health.com/blog /7-back-pain-conditions-mainly-affect -women.

Dyeo, Richard A., Sohail K. Mirza, Judith A. Turner, Brook I. Martin. "Overtreating Chronic Back Pain: Time to Back Off?" *Journal of the American Board of Family Medicine* 22 no. 1. (Jan.-Feb. 2009): 62–8. doi: 10.31/jabfm.2009 .01.080102. www.cdc.gov/mmwr/preview /mmwrhtml/mm6043a4.htm.

Fillingim, Roger B., Christopher D. King, Margaret C. Ribeiro-Dasilva, Bridgett Rahim-Williams, Joseph L. Riley, III. "Sex, Gender, and Pain: A Review of Recent Clinical and Experimental Findings." *The Journal of Pain* 10 no. 5: 447–85. www.ncbi.nlm.nih.gov/pmc/articles /PMC2677686.

Freburger, Janet K., George M. Holmes, Robert P. Agans, Anne M. Jackman, Jane D. Darter, Andrea S. Wallace, Liana D. Castel. "The Rising Prevalence of Chronic Low Back Pain." *Arch Intern Med.* 169 no. 3 (February, 2009): 251–8. doi: 10.1001/archinternmed.2008.543.

Hendry, Neil G. C. "The Hydration of the Nucleus Pulposus and Its Relation to Intervertebral Disc Derangement." (Published Feb. 1, 1958). *The Bone and Joint Journal.* Accessed Nov. 17, 2017. www.bjj.boneandjoint.org.uk/content /40-B/1/132.

"Lazy lifestyles and childhood stress inflict back pain on the young" *The Telegraph.* Accessed Nov. 18, 2017. www.telegraph.co.uk/news /health/10209066/Lazy-lifestyles-and -childhood-stress-inflict-back-pain-on-the -young.html.

Marangella, M., M. DiStefano, S. Caslis, S. Berutti, P. D'amelio, G. C. Isaia. "Effects of potassium citrate supplementation on bone metabolism." *Calcif. Tissue Int.* 74 no. 4 (April 2004): 330–5. doi: 10.1007/s00223-0030091-8.

Monrone Natalia E., Carol M. Greco, Charity G. Moore, Bruce L. Rollman, Bridget Lane, Lisa A. Morrow, Nancy Glynn, Debra K. Weiner. "A Mind-Body Program for Older Adults with Chronic Low Back Pain: A Randomized Clinical Trial." *JAMA Intern Med.* 176 no. 3 (March 2016): 329–337. doi: 10.1001 /jamainternmed.2015.803.

"Relaxation techniques: Breath control helps quell errant stress response." *Harvard Health Publishing* (updated March 18, 2016). www.health.harvard.edu/mind-and-mood /relaxation-techniques-breath-control-helps -quell-errant-stress-response.

Sebastian, Anthony, Steven T. Harris, Joan H. Ott-
away, Karen M. Todd, R. Curtis Morris, Jr. *New
England Journal of Medicine* 330 (June 1994):
1776–81. doi: 10.1001/NEJM199406233303502.

Steffens, Daniel, Chris G. Maher, Leani S. M.
Pereira, Matthew L. Stevens, Vinicius C.
Oliveira, Meredith Chapple, Luci F. Teixeira-
Salmela,Mark J. Hancock. "Prevention of
Low Back Pain: A Systematic Review and
Meta-analysis." *JAMA Intern Med.* 176 no. 2
(February 2016): 199–208. doi: 10.1001/
jamainternmed.2015.7431.

Swain, Thomas A., Gerald McGwin. "Yoga-Related
Injuries in the United States From 2001 to
2014." *Orthopaedic Journal of Sports Medicine*
4 no. 41 (Nov. 2016). doi: 10.1177/23259671703.

Wheeler, Megan S., Diane B. Arnkoff, Carol R.
Glass. "The Neuroscience of Mindfulness: How
Mindfulness Alters the Brain and Facilitates
Emotion Regulation." *Mindfulness* 8 no. 6
(Dec. 2017): 1471–87. link.springer.com
/article/10.1007/s12671-017-0742-x.

INDEX

A

Acupuncture, 138–139
Age-related degeneration, 9
Alternative therapies, 135–140
Anatomy, 4–7
Autonomic nervous system
    (ANS), 25–26

B

Backbone. *See* Spine
Back pain. *See also* Maintenance
    and prevention exercises; Pain
    relieving exercises; Strength
    and mobility exercises
    age-related degeneration, 9
    alternative therapies
        for, 135–140
    breaking bad back habits, 11
    common causes of, 9–13
    and daily life, 13–16
    depression, 13
    excess weight and
        pregnancy, 12
    and exercise therapies, 22–24

hip-related causes, 10, 12
physical trauma, 10
poor posture and
    breathing, 7–8, 12
questions to ask your
    doctor, 21
sedentary lifestyle, 12
in smokers, 13
stress, 12–13
traditional
    treatments, 19–22
travel tips for, 17
Bed rest, 21
Bent-Knee Down Dog with
    Pedal Out, 78–79
Bent-Knee Straddle
    Stretch, 86–87
Breathing
    about, 7–8, 11, 12, 17, 26
    Breathing Bridge, 68–69,
        110–111
    Breathing Bridge on
        Chair, 48–49
    Diaphragmatic Breathing with
        Legs Elevated, 36–37

Seated Posture Exercise
    with 10-Breath Breathing
    Break, 106–107, 128–129
10-Breath Breathing
    Break, 60–61
20-Breath Backward Count
    for Sleep, 64–65
Breathing Bridge, 68–69, 110–111
Breathing Bridge on
    Chair, 48–49

C

Cat Flow, 54–55, 122–123
Cervical vertebrae, 4
Child's Pose, 40–41
Child's Pose with Reach, 58–59
Chiropractic care, 138
Cobra, 74–75
Coccyx, 4
Cognitive behavioral therapy
    (CBT), 139–140
Compassion Meditation, 130–132
Cook, Gray, 101
Crura, 7

D

Degenerative breakdown, 9
Dehydration, 17
Depression, 11, 13
Diaphragm, 7–8
Diaphragmatic Breathing with
    Legs Elevated, 36–37
Disc herniation, 10, 20
Discs, 5
Dominant-side
    tendencies, 13–14, 25
Driving, 15
Dry needling, 138

E

Equipment, 32
Erector spinae muscles, 7
Ergonomics, 15
Exercise. See also Maintenance
    and prevention exercises; Pain-
    relieving exercises; Strength
    and mobility exercises
    about the exercises, 29–32
    equipment needed, 32
    as self-care, 22–24
    vs. traditional treatments, 19–20
Extension, 5, 6
Extensor muscles, 6–7

F

Fascia, 137
Fight-or-flight
    response, 12–13, 25–26
Flexion, 5, 6

Flexor muscles, 7
Flowing Bridge, 88–89
Flowing Chair Squat, 120–121
Foam rollers, 137
Fractures, 10

G

Gait mechanics, 112–114
Gate Pose, 52–53
Gluteal muscles (glutes), 7

H

Hip flexors, 7, 17
Hip problems, 10, 12
Household chores, 14–15
Hydration, 17

I

Imaging scans, 19–20, 21
Intramuscular stimulation
    (IMS), 138

K

Kneeling Lunge, 50–51
Kneeling Lunge with
    Reach, 98–99
Kyphotic curvature, 6

L

Lateral movement, 6
Laxity, 12
Legs Up the Wall, 38–39, 126–127

Lifting, 15
Ligaments, 5–6, 9
Locust, 96–97
Lordotic curvature, 6
Lumbar vertebrae, 4–5, 7

M

Maintenance and
    prevention exercises
    about, 109
    Breathing Bridge, 110–111
    Cat Flow, 122–123
    Compassion
        Meditation, 130–132
    Flowing Chair Squat, 120–121
    Legs Up the Wall, 126–127
    Seated Posture Exercise
        with 10-Breath Breathing
        Break, 128–129
    Supine Single-Leg, Bent-Knee
        Twist, 118–119
    Supported Back-Release
        Squat, 124–125
    Walking with Awareness of Gait
        Mechanics, 112–114
    Warrior Hip Flexor
        Stretch, 116–117
Massage Therapy, 137
Meditation
    Compassion Meditation, 130–132
    mindfulness meditation, 139
Mind-body connection, 24–26.
    See also Breathing
Mindfulness meditation, 139
Mood disorders, 13
Muscles, 6–7

N

Narcotic prescriptions, 19, 21, 22
90/90 Seated Twist, 100–101

O

Oblique muscles, 7
Opioids, 19, 21, 22
Over-the-counter medications, 22

P

Pain-relieving exercises
 about, 35
 Breathing Bridge on
  Chair, 48–49
 Cat Flow, 54–55
 Child's Pose, 40–41
 Child's Pose with Reach, 58–59
 Diaphragmatic Breathing with
  Legs Elevated, 36–37
 Gate Pose, 52–53
 Kneeling Lunge, 50–51
 Legs Up the Wall, 38–39
 Progressive Muscle
  Relaxation, 62–63
 Seated Figure-Four Hip
  Opener, 42–43
 Supine Figure-Four
  Stretch, 56–57
 Supported Back-Release
  Squat, 46–47
 Supported Warrior Hip Flexor
  Stretch, 44–45
 10-Breath Breathing
  Break, 60–61

 20-Breath Backward Count
  for Sleep, 64–65
Parasympathetic nervous
 system, 25–26
Pharmaceuticals, 19, 22
Physical therapy (PT), 21, 135
Physical trauma, 10
Pigeon, 102–103
Pilates, 136
Piriformis syndrome, 10, 12
Posture, 11, 12
Pregnancy, 12
Progressive Muscle
 Relaxation, 62–63
Psoas major muscle, 7–8

Q

Quadrates lumborum (QL)
 muscles, 7

R

Recreation and sports, 16
Relaxation
 Progressive Muscle
  Relaxation, 62–63
Rest and repose response, 25
Rib cage, 7–8
Roll-Into-a-Ball Core
 Exercise, 72–73
Rotation, 6, 30

S

Sacroiliac (SI) joints, 10
Sacrum, 4, 10

Sciatic nerve, 12
Seated Bent-Knee
 Twist, 76–77
Seated Figure-Four Hip
 Opener, 42–43
Seated Hamstring and Hip
 Stretch, 104–105
Seated Posture Exercise
 with 10-Breath Breathing
 Break, 106–107, 128–129
Sedentary lifestyles, 12
Segmented Forearm
 Plank, 92–93
Self-care, 11, 22–24
Self-myofascial release
 (SMR), 137
Side Forearm Plank, 94–95
Sitting, 17
Sleeping
 and back pain, 15–16
 20-Breath Backward Count
  for Sleep, 64–65
Slumping, 11
Smoking, 13
Sphinx with Head
 Turns, 70–71
Spinal cord, 4, 9
Spinal osteoarthritis, 9
Spine
 anatomy of, 4–6
 how breathing impacts, 7–8
 muscles that support
  and move, 6–7
Spondylolisthesis, 9
Standing, 17
Standing Side Bend, 80–81
Stenosis, 9, 20

Strength and mobility exercises
about, 67
Bent-Knee Down Dog with
Pedal Out, 78–79
Bent-Knee Straddle
Stretch, 86–87
Breathing Bridge, 68–69
Cobra, 74–75
Flowing Bridge, 88–89
Kneeling Lunge with
Reach, 98–99
Locust, 96–97
90/90 Seated Twist, 100–101
Pigeon, 102–103
Roll-Into-a-Ball Core
Exercise, 72–73
Seated Bent-Knee Twist, 76–77
Seated Hamstring and Hip
Stretch, 104–105
Seated Posture Exercise
with 10-Breath Breathing
Break, 106–107
Segmented Forearm
Plank, 92–93
Side Forearm Plank, 94–95
Sphinx with Head Turns, 70–71
Standing Side Bend, 80–81

Supine Double Bent-Knee
Twist, 82–83
Supine Figure-Four
Twist, 84–85
Windmill Twist, 90–91
Stress, 12–13, 26
Stretching, 17, 29–30
Supine Double Bent-Knee
Twist, 82–83
Supine Figure-Four
Stretch, 56–57
Supine Figure-Four Twist, 84–85
Supine Single-Leg, Bent-Knee
Twist, 118–119
Supported Back-Release Squat,
46–47, 124–125
Supported Warrior Hip Flexor
Stretch, 44–45
Surgery, 20, 21
Sympathetic nervous
system, 25–26

T

Tai chi, 136
10-Breath Breathing
Break, 60–61

Thoracic vertebrae, 4–5
Travel, 15, 17
T-spine (thoracic spine), 14
20-Breath Backward Count for
Sleep, 64–65
Twisting, 14, 67. *See also* Strength
and mobility exercises

V

Vertebrae, 4

W

Walking with Awareness of Gait
Mechanics, 112–114
Warrior Hip Flexor
Stretch, 116–117
Weight, 12
Windmill Twist, 90–91
Work/screen time, 15

Y

Yoga, 135–136

ACKNOWLEDGMENTS

As much as I'm extremely passionate about helping people breathe, move, and feel better in their bodies and lives, writing a book about back pain was not initially part of my plan this year. It was only after Callisto reached out to me after reading articles I'd written on the topic, making a convincing pitch for why the world needed a book on practical back pain solutions and why I was the one to write it, that I realized I needed to make it happen. I'm extremely grateful to Callisto for believing in me!

I'm also grateful to my publisher for teaming me with my primary editor and master hand-holder, Susan Randol, who got me through this project within a tight deadline, despite all the headaches of my travel schedule, having to evacuate for a hurricane, and dealing with the loss of a four-legged family member. Thank you, Susan, for all your support and encouragement.

I also want to acknowledge my editors at CNN Health, David Allan and Jamie Gumbrecht. Over the past few years of writing for them, they've helped me find my voice and given me the confidence to share my experiences and advice on a worldwide platform.

Without an understanding of how correcting movement patterns can alleviate pain, I wouldn't have been able to write this book. Early in my career I was lucky enough to read *Athletic Body in Balance* by Gray Cook, creator of the Functional Movement Systems. The book introduced me to the potential of corrective exercises. And Gray has continued to motivate and inspire me now that I've had the chance to get to know him personally and have had the privilege of sharing the stage with him at Perform Better Summit events.

Throughout this book, I drive home the significance of breathing optimally. I have Ron Hruska and the Postural Restoration Institute™ (PRI) to thank for teaching me that breathing is arguably our most fundamental movement pattern.

Specifically, I want to thank Mike Cantrell for taking extra time to help me understand complex PRI concepts, and James Anderson for inspiring me to share the power of breathing biomechanics with the world in the most practical, understandable ways possible.

In the introduction, I mention my personal experience with back pain and the progressive doctor from the Toronto Blue Jays, who helped me during my second acute injury. He demonstrated the efficacy of alternatives to narcotics and bed rest. Thank you, Dr. Nishin Tambay!

I also want to thank Dr. Tim Bain, the team chiropractor for the Tampa Bay Lightning, who showed me how back pain treatment could be more effective through an integrative approach that includes not only my mobility and restorative exercises, but also chiropractic, physical therapy, and massage.

No book is ever written without the support and love of friends and family. For that reason, I want to thank one of my best friends, Suzanne Poitras, who not only served as a supportive friend but also as my attorney in reviewing my book contract. I'm so blessed to have you in my life, Suzanne. And to my friend Christina Chatfield, although we didn't see each other much during this process because I was buried with work, I knew you were there if I needed you, and I appreciate the quick walks you took with me to help clear my head now and then.

To my beautiful, amazing daughter Amanda, you have always made me feel like I was the best writer you knew, asking my opinion on anything you wrote and running all of your blog posts by me for editing. Whenever I hit a sticking point in this project, I remembered your confidence in me. How could I not finish this if my daughter believes in me? I love you so much, Ladybug.

And to my two awesome sons Ryan and Luke: You both inspire me to want to be better and do better in the world. I'm so proud of you both.

Anyone who knows me well would not be surprised that I have to thank my dogs. Any time I sat at my desk, they were at my feet or trying to climb into my lap, looking for attention. That probably doesn't sound helpful. Admittedly, it was a little distracting at times, but it's also highly motivating to be surrounded by the wagging tails of unconditional love. The dog people reading this definitely understand.

Last, but certainly never least, I want to thank my husband for being my biggest supporter, motivator, and head cheerleader. Donovan, you are my favorite human. You make me a better person and inspire me to want to do more for others—like writing this book to help people get out of pain. I could undoubtedly write an entire book just explaining how loving you has positively changed the course of my life. Maybe, someday, I will . . .

ABOUT THE AUTHOR

Dana Santas, CSCS, E-RYT is a mind-body coach in professional sports, the yoga expert for *CNN Health*, and an international speaker/presenter on ways to help people breathe, move, feel better in their bodies, and be happier and healthier in their lives. Known as the "Mobility Maker," she has more than 13 years of experience working with over 40 professional sports teams and hundreds of athletes in Major League Baseball (MLB), the National Hockey League (NHL), the National Basketball Association (NBA), the National Football League (NFL), the Professional Golfers' Association (PGA), the Women's Tennis Association (WTA), and World Wrestling Entertainment (WWE). Additionally, she trains veterans and tactical professionals, and is proud to have served as the yoga coach to the Boston Fire Department.

As a fitness expert, Dana is a regular guest on shows like *Daytime TV*, *BayNews 9*, and *Good Morning Tampa Bay*. As a writer, she has done interviews and articles for more than 100 media outlets, including *Sports Illustrated*, *Dr. Oz The Good Life*, *Men's Health*, *Prevention*, *Shape*, *Success*, *Oxygen*, Fox Sports, CNN, and more.

Dana earned her BA cum laude/with honors from Tufts University. Specializing in integrative mobility, functional movement, and breathing biomechanics, Dana is a certified strength and conditioning coach through the National Strength & Conditioning Association (NSCA) and has received extensive education through the Postural Restoration Institute™ (PRI), as well as certifications with Titleist Performance Institute (TPI), Functional Movement Systems (FMS, FRC, SFMA), the American College of Sports Medicine (ACSM), and the National Academy of Sports Medicine (NASM). An experienced registered yoga teacher (E-RYT) and educator, she continually hones her skills and expertise through research, coursework, and by learning from the professional sports team coaches, trainers, therapists, and doctors she has the privilege to work alongside on an ongoing basis.

The lucky mother of three amazing children (and two rescue pups), Dana lives in the Tampa Bay area with her very best friend and love of her life, her husband Donovan.

You can learn more about Dana's work at www.MobilityMaker.com and connect with her on social media: @MobilityMaker on Facebook, Instagram, and Twitter.

CPSIA information can be obtained
at www.ICGtesting.com
Printed in the USA
BVOW10s1417231217
503487BV00005B/6/P